PORTRAIT OF A FITNESS FANATIC

MARK OMAN
Illustrations by
GARY PATTERSON

A THOUGHT FACTORY BOOK

CONTEMPORARY
BOOKS, INC.
CHICAGO

Library of Congress Cataloging in Publication Data

Oman, Mark.
Portrait of a fitness fanatic.

1. Exercise—Anecdotes, facetiae, satire, etc.
2. Physical fitness—Anecdotes, facetiae, satire, etc.
I. Title.
PN6231.E9845 1985 818'.5402 85-5901
ISBN 0-8092-5254-6

Published by Contemporary Books, Inc.
180 North Michigan Avenue, Chicago, Illinois 60601
Manufactured in the United States of America
Library of Congress Catalog Card Number: 85-5901
International Standard Book Number: 0-8092-5254-6

Published simultaneously in Canada by Beaverbooks, Ltd.
195 Allstate Parkway, Valleywood Business Park
Markham, Ontario L3R 4T8 Canada

Published by arrangement with the Thought Factory
P.O. Box 5515, Sherman Oaks, CA 91413

For my dearest wife, Barbara . . .

Who for ten years has dedicated her life to physical fitness; has committed herself to only the healthiest eating habits, sharing with me the nutritional delights of yogurt and wheat germ waffles for breakfast, chile con tofu for lunch, seaweed salad and spaghetti with turkey balls for dinner, and carob chip whip for dessert . . .

For all the good and right and healthy ways she has taught me these ten long years, I say with all my heart . . . "How 'bout a pork chop once in a while!"

CONTENTS

INTRODUCTION

In Perspiring Pursuit of the Body Beautiful

Fitness Fanatics—they are out there by the millions! Many of your friends and neighbors may, in fact, be card-carrying members of the "no pain, no gain" fitness fraternity. The fact that they look no more fit than they look like Morgan Brittany or Tom Selleck has nothing to do with it. To many a Fitness Fanatic, a positive mental attitude about exercising is the same as actually doing it. This may explain why some fitness enthusiasts tell you "the body is the temple of the soul"—even when theirs look more like the Leaning Tower of Too Much Pizza.

But let's face it, everyone wants a gorgeous, desirable, sexy body, preferably their own.

From there, it is just a hop, skip, and $75 for a pair of high performance footgear and the novice Fitness Fanatic is off and running to tank tops, tofu burgers, and their neighborhood fitness spa. They're on the exercise treadmill.

While the Fitness Fanatics you are about to meet on the following pages may not always be perfect physical specimens, they are, each and every one, forever in perspiring pursuit of The Body Beautiful.

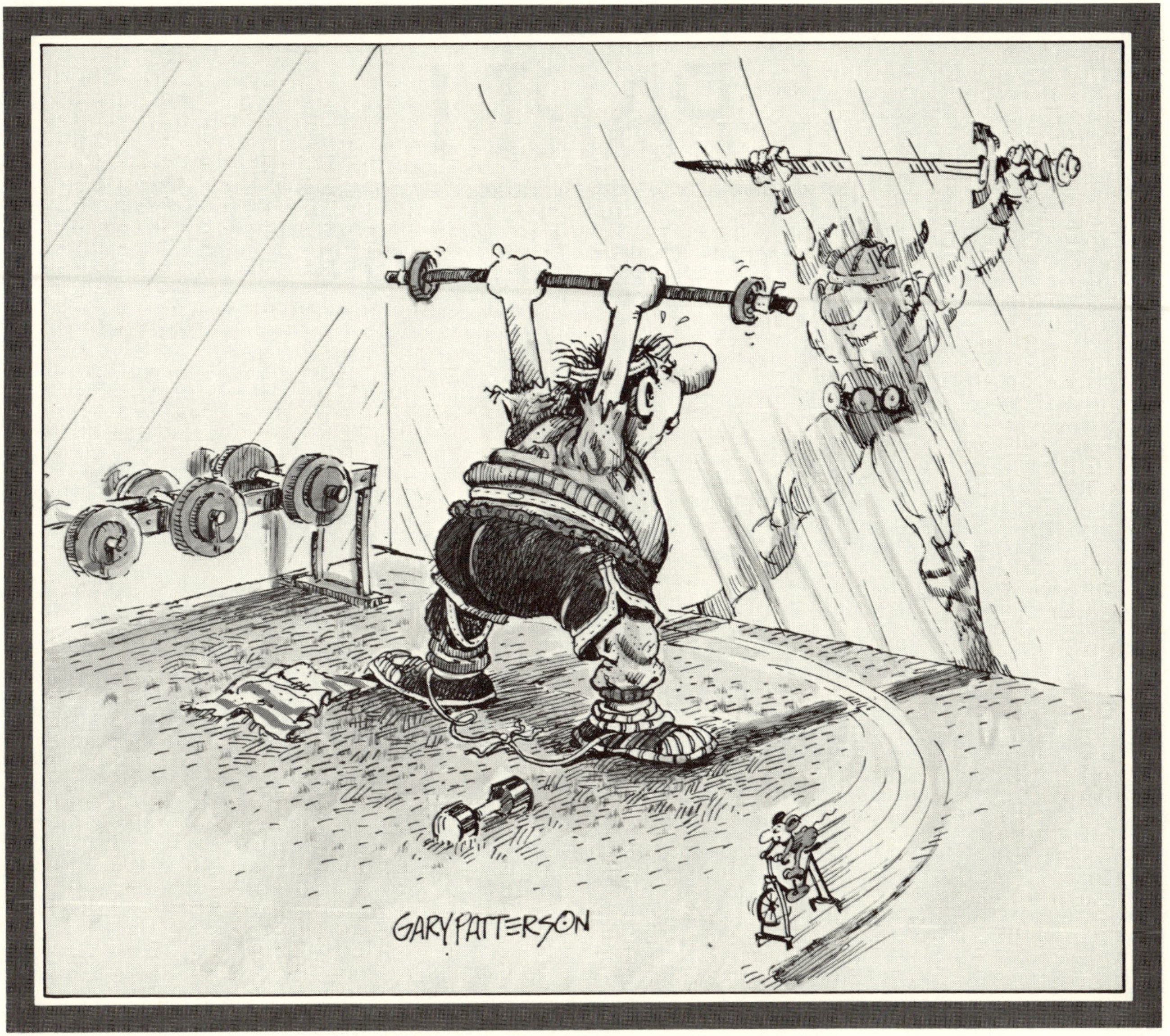

THE BODY BEAUTIFUL

PART I

Aerobic Animals

During the last few years, aerobic exercise has become so popular that thousands of people who spent years trying to squeeze into jogging suits with the sole intention of being fashionable, are now actually wearing them in 10K races, 26-mile marathons, and mind-boggling 100-mile ultra marathons.

And it's not just runners: Former pool paddlers are training for ocean crossings, and cyclists who just abandoned their training wheels are gearing up for coast-to-coast pedal pushing. These Aerobic Animals go beyond mere fitness. Their attitude is: "If running two miles a day is going to make me healthy, then just imagine what running a hundred miles across the Sierras will do!"

1

LOOSENING UP

Before engaging in any workout, the Aerobic Animal always allows time for loosening up and stretching. Some types of stretching are more beneficial than others. Things like toe touching, hurdler's stretch, sit-ups, and the like have recently been shown to be over-rated and even dangerous—thank goodness!

On the other hand, a safe and positive exercise is standing on your tippy tippy toes and reaching way back into the top pantry shelf, stretching fingertips behind the sugar frosted flakes until they grasp onto the three-pound bag of Famous Amos Chocolate Chip Cookies. Now the stretching has a meaningful and delicious purpose.

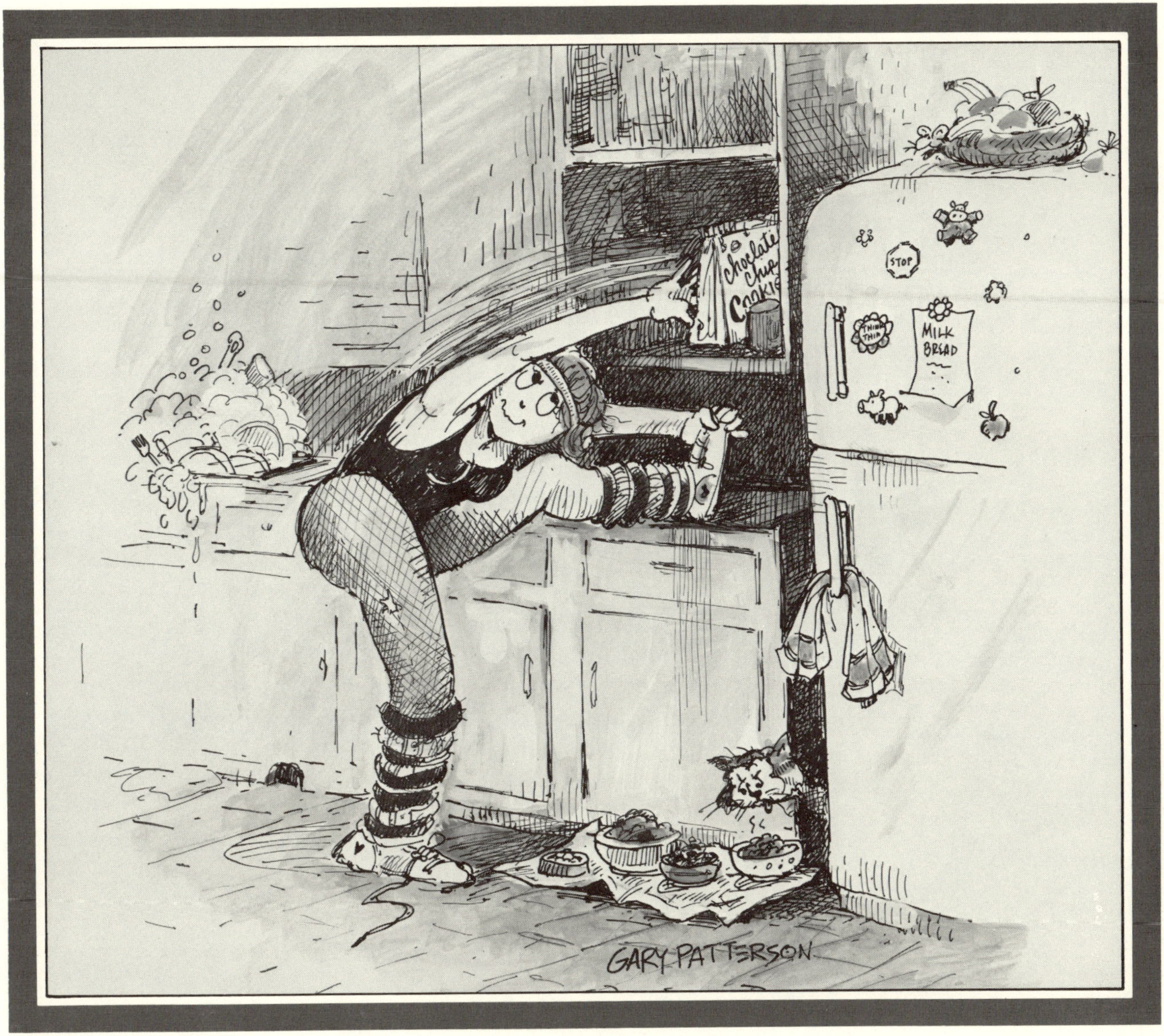

STRETCHING

2

BECAUSE *YOU* WANT TO DO IT!

Once Aerobic Animals are loose and limber, they are ready to begin an extended workout. The serious minded are careful about weighing the many types of aerobic exercises before committing themselves. Or being committed.

One of the most common reasons people give up on exercise programs is boredom. So, remember to choose something that's fun, something you'll be able to do and enjoy for the rest of your life—even if it's shortened.

Sex is good. Don't do it because your doctor says it's good for you, or because your spouse wants you to, or your neighbor says that's what friends are for, but because *you* want to do it.

When should you do it? One study shows that of those who engage in sex—as an aerobic exercise—in the morning before work, 79% stayed with it. Of those who made it a standing habit on their lunch hour, 50% hung in there. But of those who tried to squeeze it in after work before going home, only 25% were able to make it a regular affair . . . and they didn't live long enough to enjoy it.

3

HAPPY FEET, WHY ARE YOU BLUE?

Do you like your feet?

Come on now. The truth.

The fact is your feet already have a lot going against them, but when the tenderfoot Fitness Fanatic jumps into aerobic exercise, it is usually head over heels, feet first. Why leave it up to them? What have they ever done for you? Anything with 38 muscles, 52 bones, and 214 ligaments doesn't have a lot of room for smarts. But they do have feelings and they can be easily hurt.

So when you engage in aerobic exercise and your feet hurt, even the slightest, it's their way of saying: "Take a load off—enough is enough!"

Remember, listen to your feet!

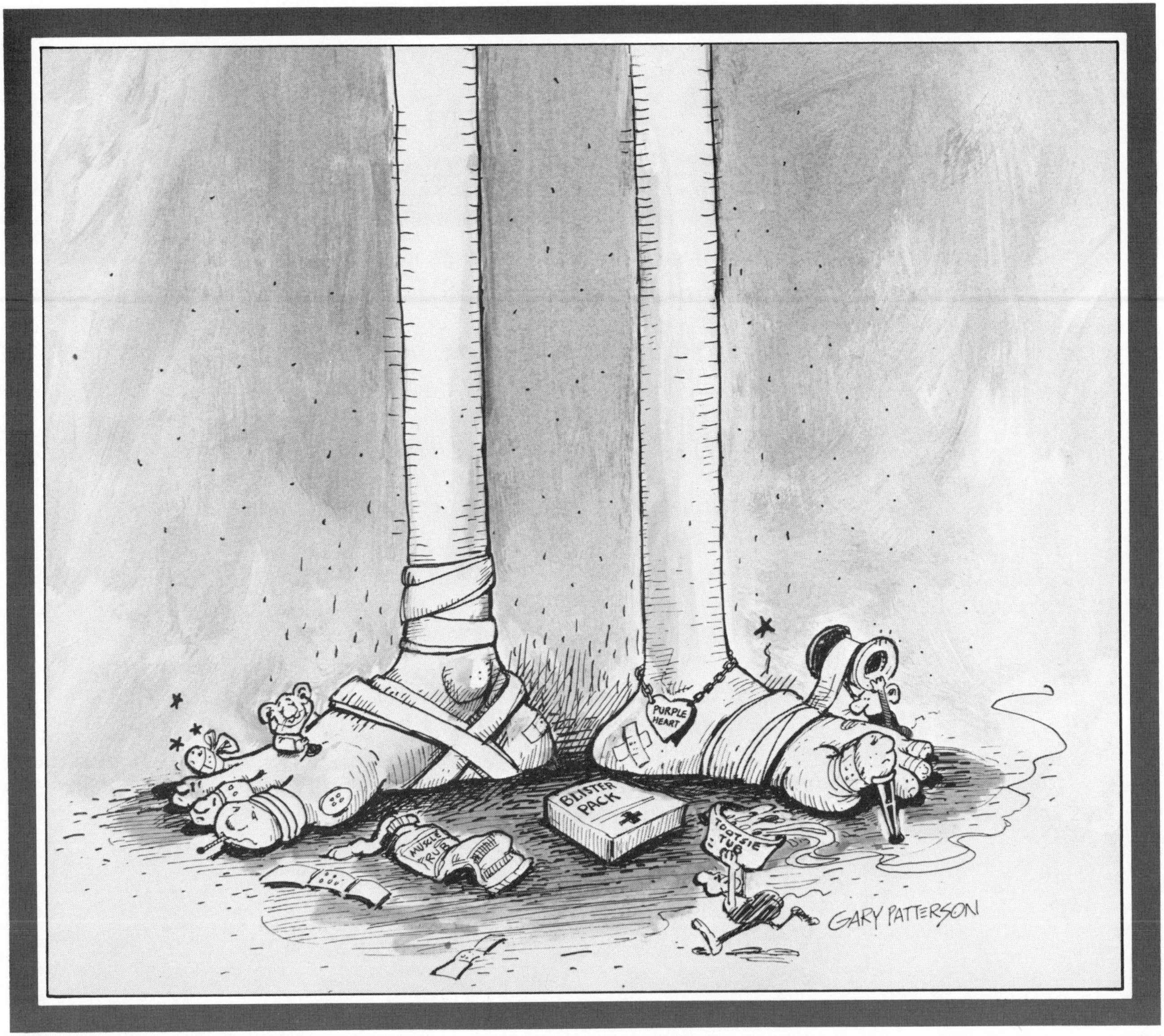

RUNNERS FEET

4

A WALK ON THE WILD SIDE

One form of aerobic exercise that nearly everyone is capable of doing is walking forward.

There's nothing quite like a long, brisk walk in the woods to open up those sinuses, clear out that old catch-all closet between the ears, and make you appreciate what a terrific person you really are. After all, where else can you find such good company and brilliant conversation?

And then we have race walking. Aerobic Animals who willingly engage in race walking have the heart of a lion and the pluck of a duck!

Heralded by some devotees as the best cardiovascular exercise in the world, race walking is virtually injury free—that is, from the walking itself. The bad news is that when your hips and elbows swivel and swing madly from stem to stern, you look like a duck whose Fruit of the Loom has been invaded by the fleas of a thousand camels.

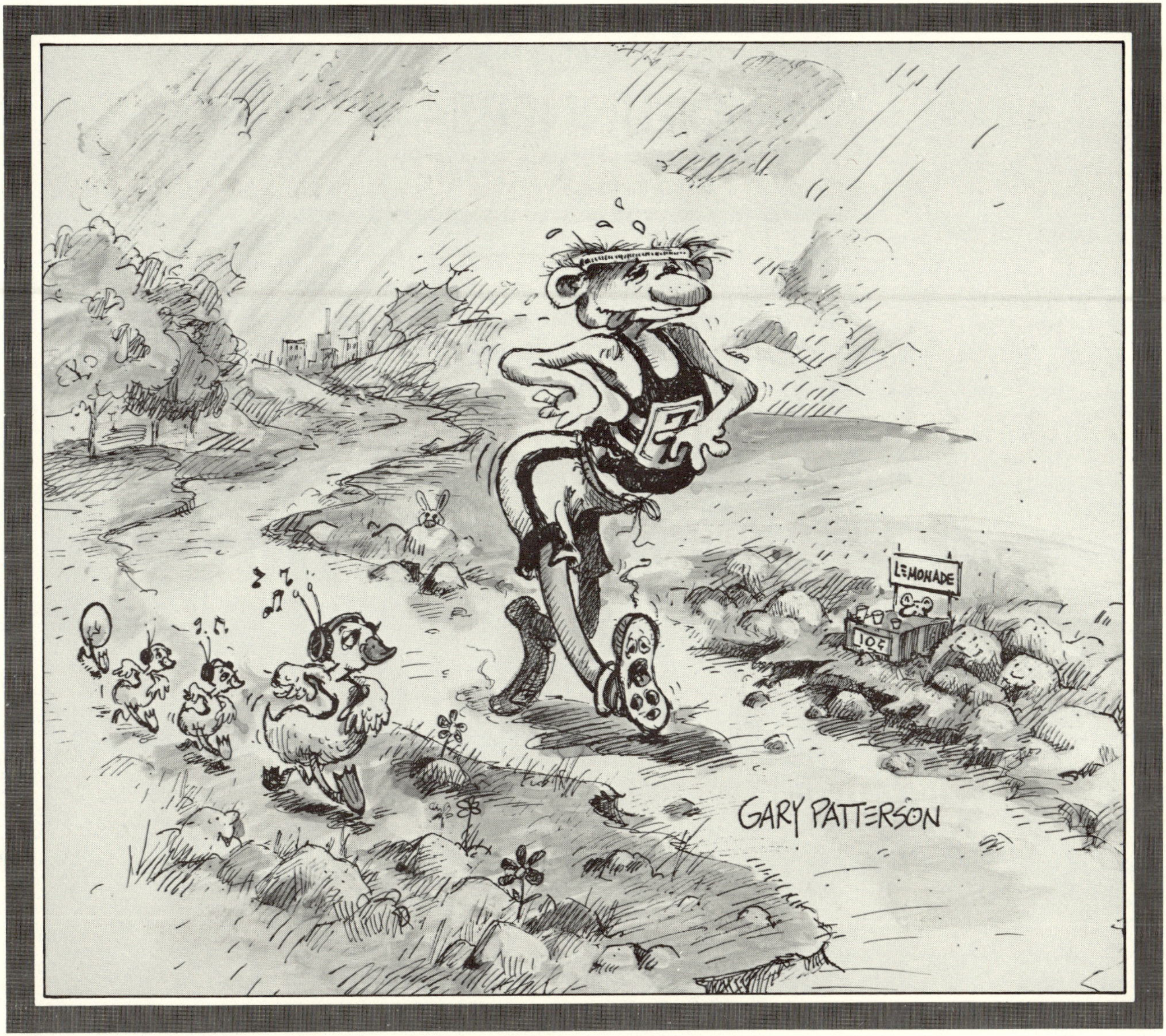

THE RACE WALKER

5

JOGGERS vs. RUNNERS— A BREED APART

It is of paramount importance to understand the difference between jogging and running. Therein lies the difference between a trot around the block and galloping down the hot asphalt to Boston!

Though some argue that jogging and running are interchangeable terms for the same exercise, don't be misled. Joggers are often only interested in fashion. They either look incredibly bored or are wearing headphones and getting it on with Michael Jackson, regardless of gender.

What type are you?

WHAT TYPE ARE YOU?

Joggers	Runners
Like people, have lots of friends, and are fun to be around	Have one and only one meaningful relationship—with their shoes.
Are happy to survive their daily trots and still be able to bend over and untie their laces.	Aren't happy unless they put in their daily ten miles of roadwork and feel as though they've been through the Spanish Inquisition.
Drive bigger, older automobiles or antique sports cars that never seem to run on all cylinders—very much like their owners.	Drive economical cars that run forever on a teaspoonful of fuel.

Sprinters prefer turbo-charged wheels. They love to blow them out on straightaways—when they're not in the shop having their engines rebuilt, also like their owners.

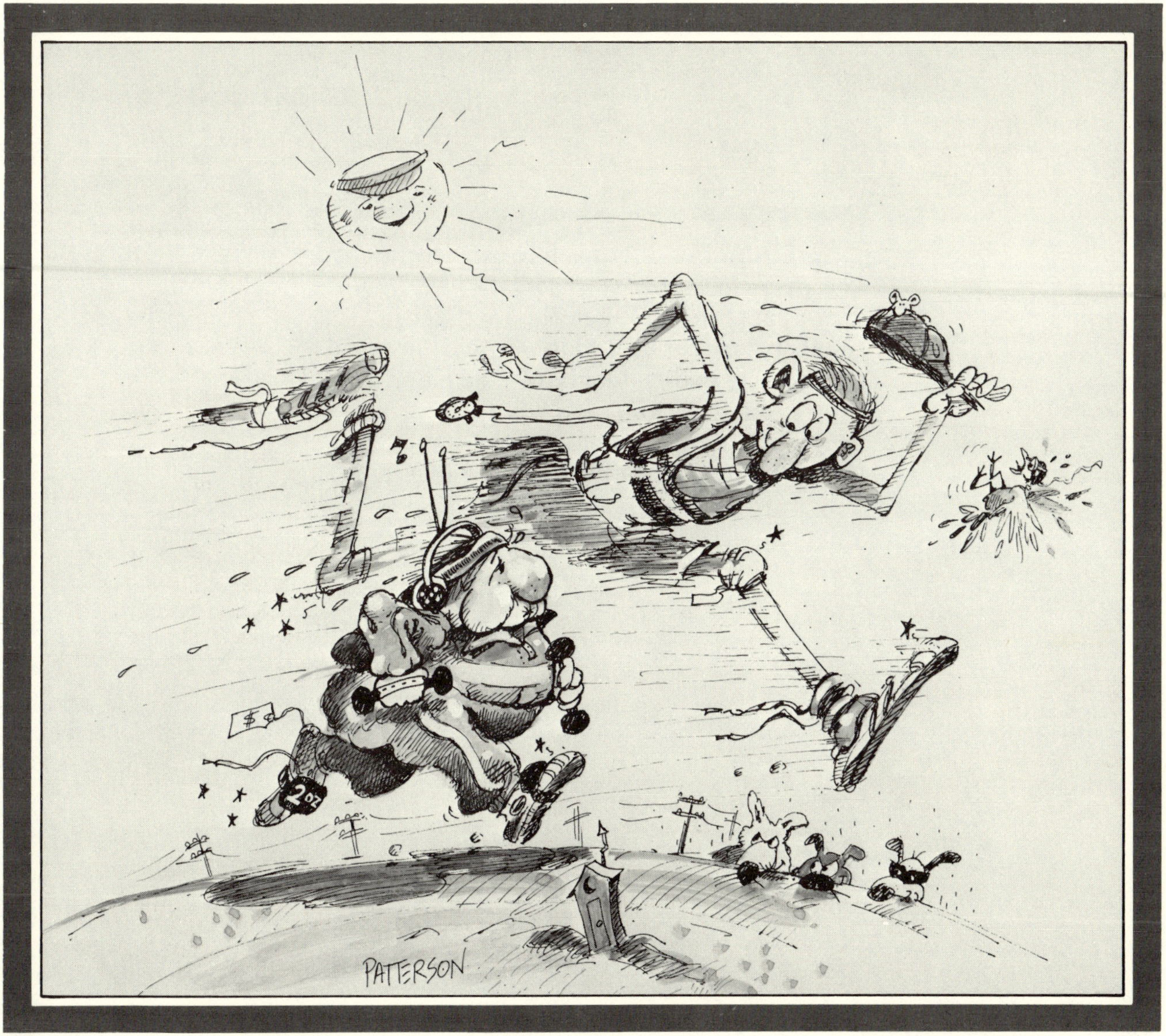

THE SPRINTER

Once running fanatics have vowed fidelity to a particular pair of shoes, it's usually until death parts them. When the road gets rougher, lonelier and tougher, and the wind gets colder, and suddenly they're older, they prefer to patch things up with rubberized goop than to throw away all the good years they and their shoes have shared together.

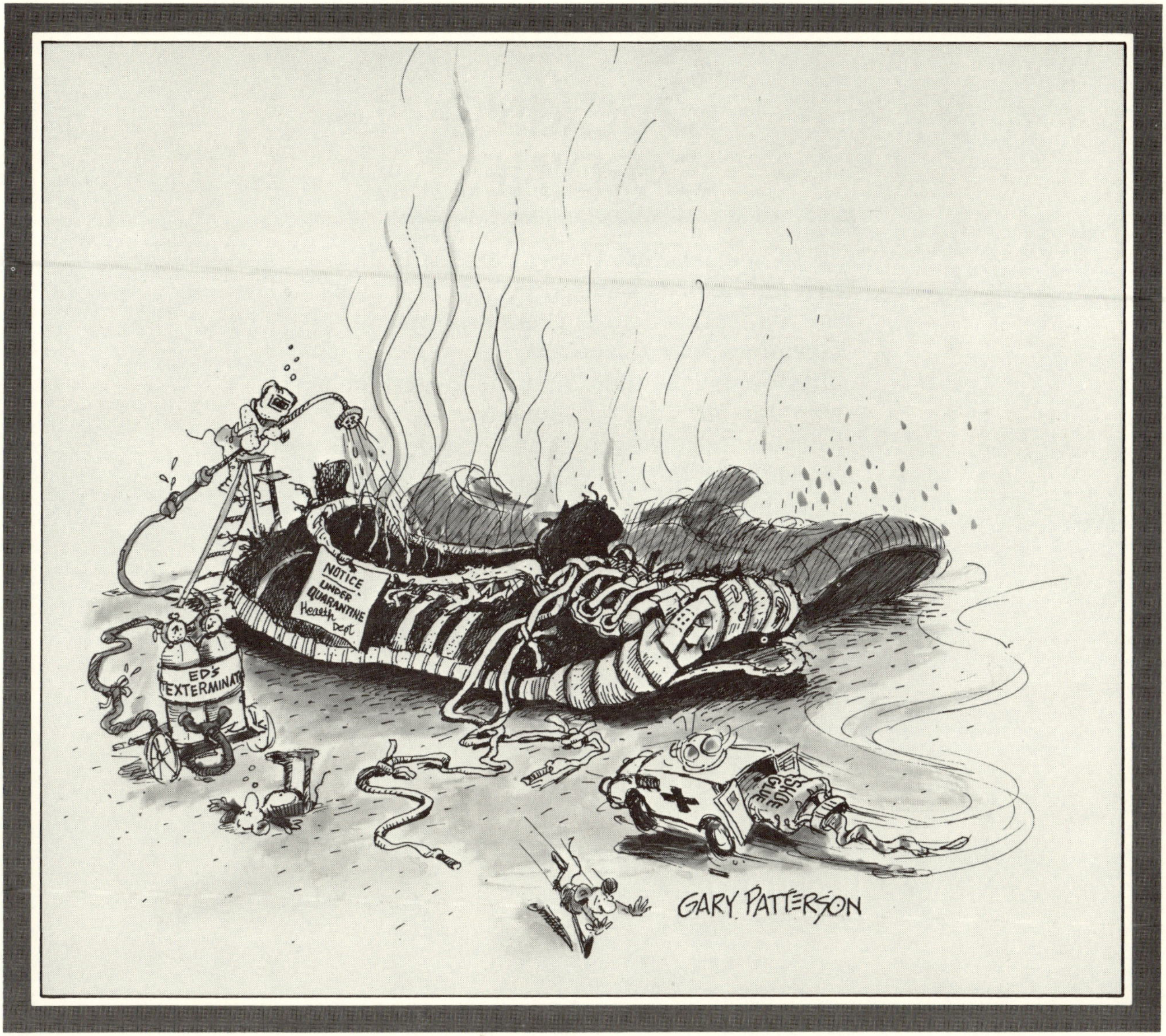
NOTICE
UNDER QUARANTINE
Health Dept
ED's EXTERMINAT
SHOE GLUE
GARY PATTERSON

6

Sucking Sardines

If the purpose of aerobic exercise is to burn up the body's stored fat, it's also true that your fat content is precisely what determines your floatability.

It must follow, then, that the longer you swim, the more fat you burn up. Unfortunately, the more fat burned up, the less you have to keep you afloat. The longer you swim and the more fit you become, the closer you are to drowning. This is known simply as sucking sardines.

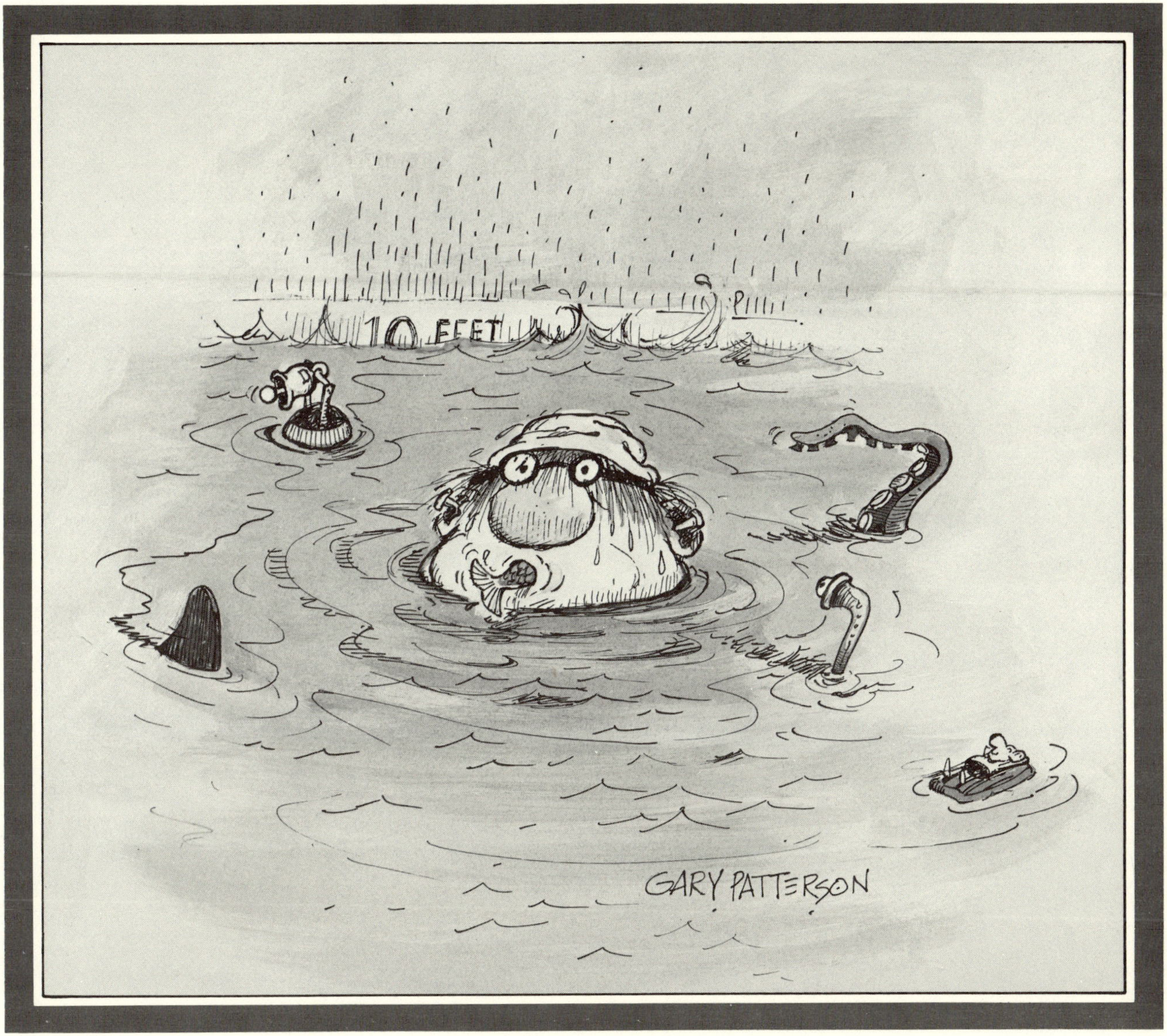

THE SWIMMER

7

THE PASSIONATE PEDAL-PUSHER

Pedal-pushing fanatics think of themselves as members of an elite two-wheeled cavalry. Whether alone, or riding in formations with the rest of the troops, passionate pedal-pushers always seem to be on their way to somewhere important.

They seem fearless but actually have a few wheels missing.

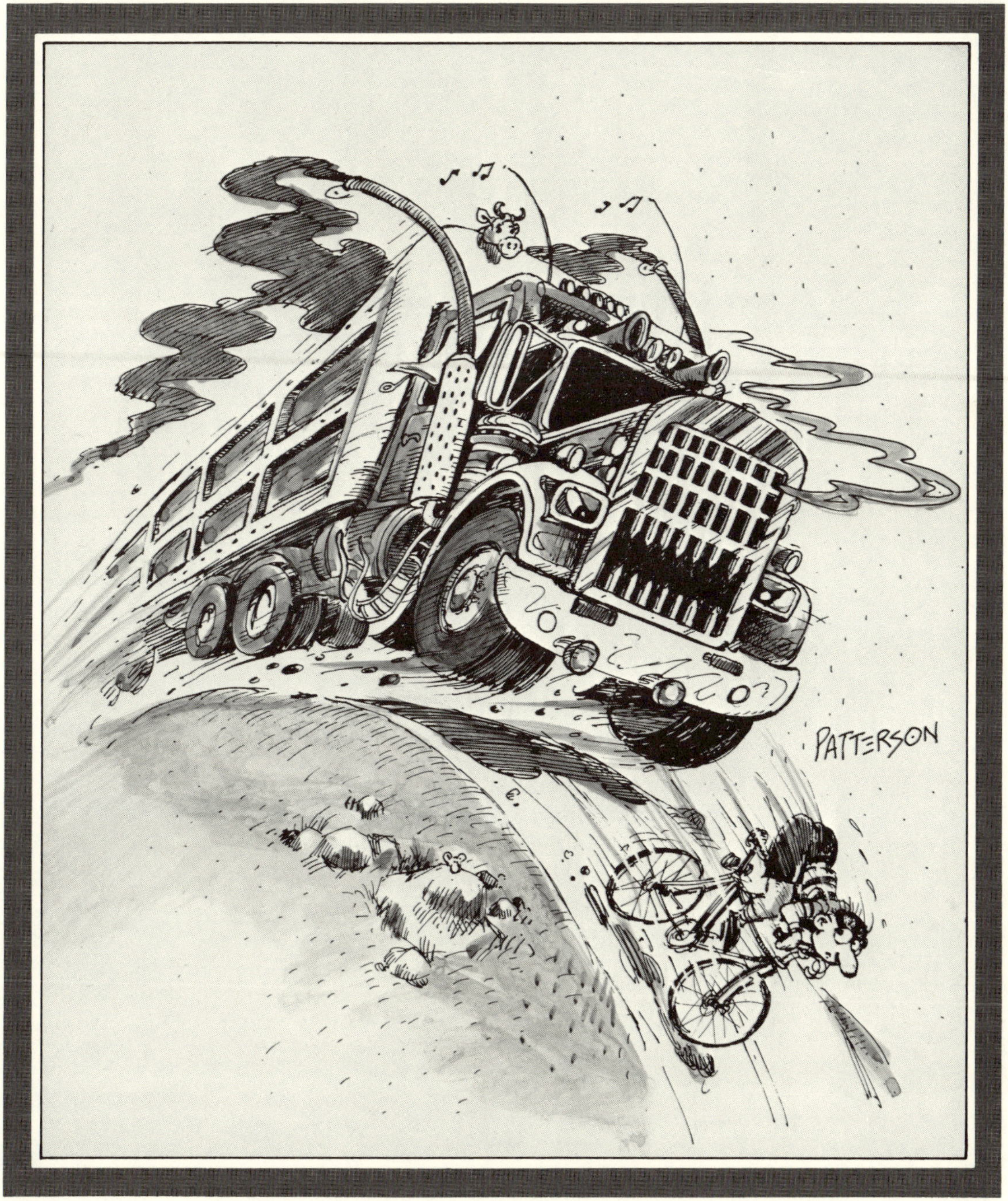

PUSHING IT

REAL PEDAL-PUSHING FANATICS:

- Have thighs like giant Sequoias. They have thick trunks and bark when approached.
- Are always in training. Even when they are not riding, they walk around like the Hunchback of Notre Dame, their shirts stuffed with bottles of Gatorade and bags of complex carbohydrates.
- Wear a chamois on the inside of their shorts to cushion the ride.
- Are protective about their wheels. They take them everywhere: to the office, to the executive washroom, to church, and to the savings and loan where they mortgaged their house to buy the thing.

For the truly gourmand cyclist with epicurean tastes, nothing can satisfy like a 12-speed Italian Cannelloni with Fettuccine frame, Aldente stem and handlebars, Antipasto forks, Scallopini seat, Ricotta rims, and Rigatoni special tubing.

Grab the chianti and go for it!

8

TRIATHLETES

The men and women who take part in Triathlons are not well. The best thing we can all do is ignore them and maybe they'll run away.

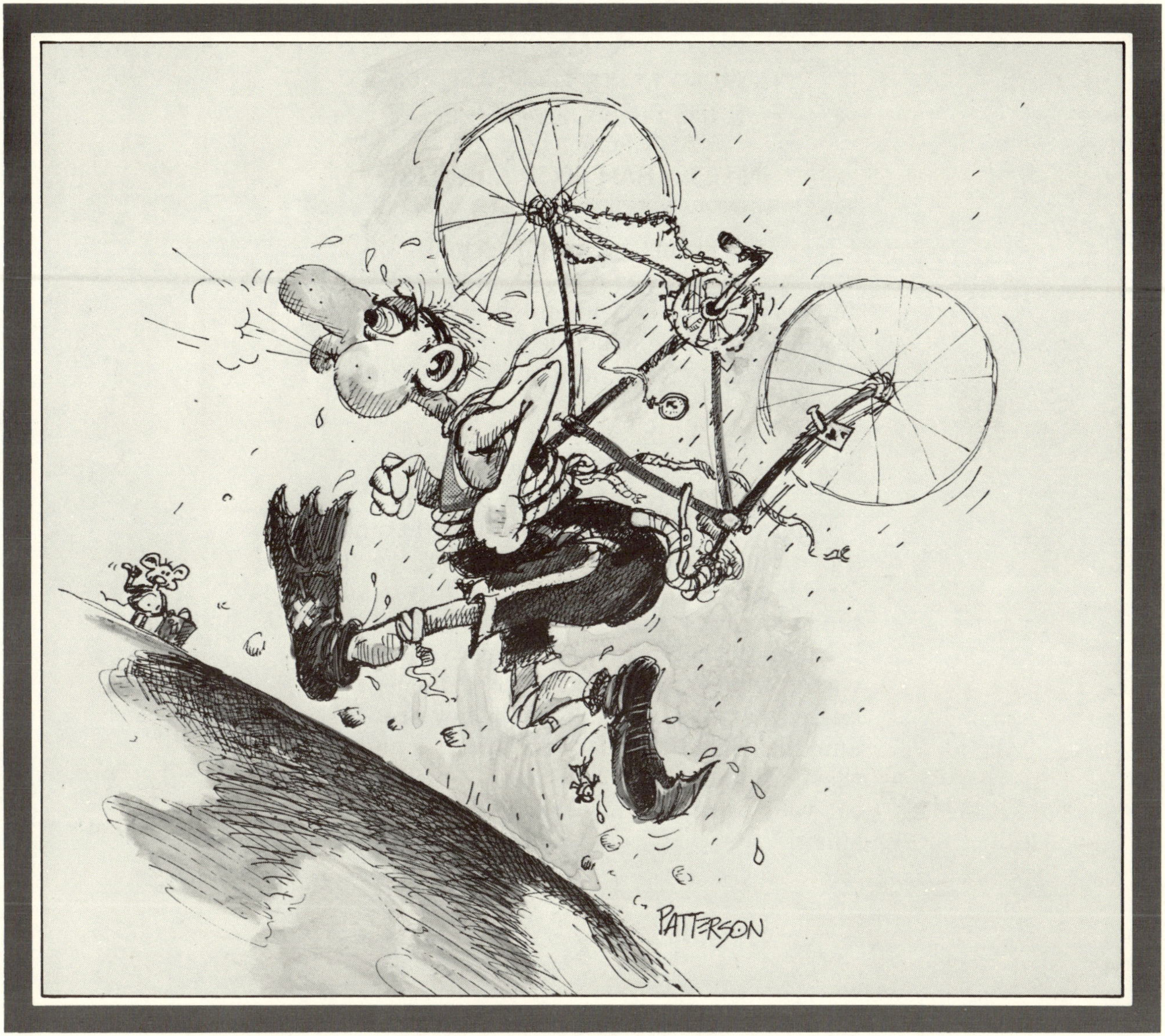

THE TRIATHLETE

9
DANCE AEROBICS
-OR-
HOW TO MAKE A LINEBACKER FOR THE PITTSBURGH STEELERS BEG FOR MERCY IN LESS THAN SIXTY MINUTES

More than nineteen million Americans are now hooked on some form of dance exercise, and it is primarily women who are the most susceptible to its seductive allure.

Whichever one of the many trade names it comes disguised under, the activity is masochistic. At the end of a particularly good workout, you can hear cries of . . .

"It hurts! It hurts! God, I love it!"

Before getting all lathered up and doing something your body may never forgive you for, take a few minutes and carefully read the following:

No matter what they may tell you, the women who engage in hard-core dance exercise are not your friends. They are animals! Give them fifty-six minutes and they will go for your throat . . . your thighs . . . your tummy, fanny, heart, mind, and spirit!

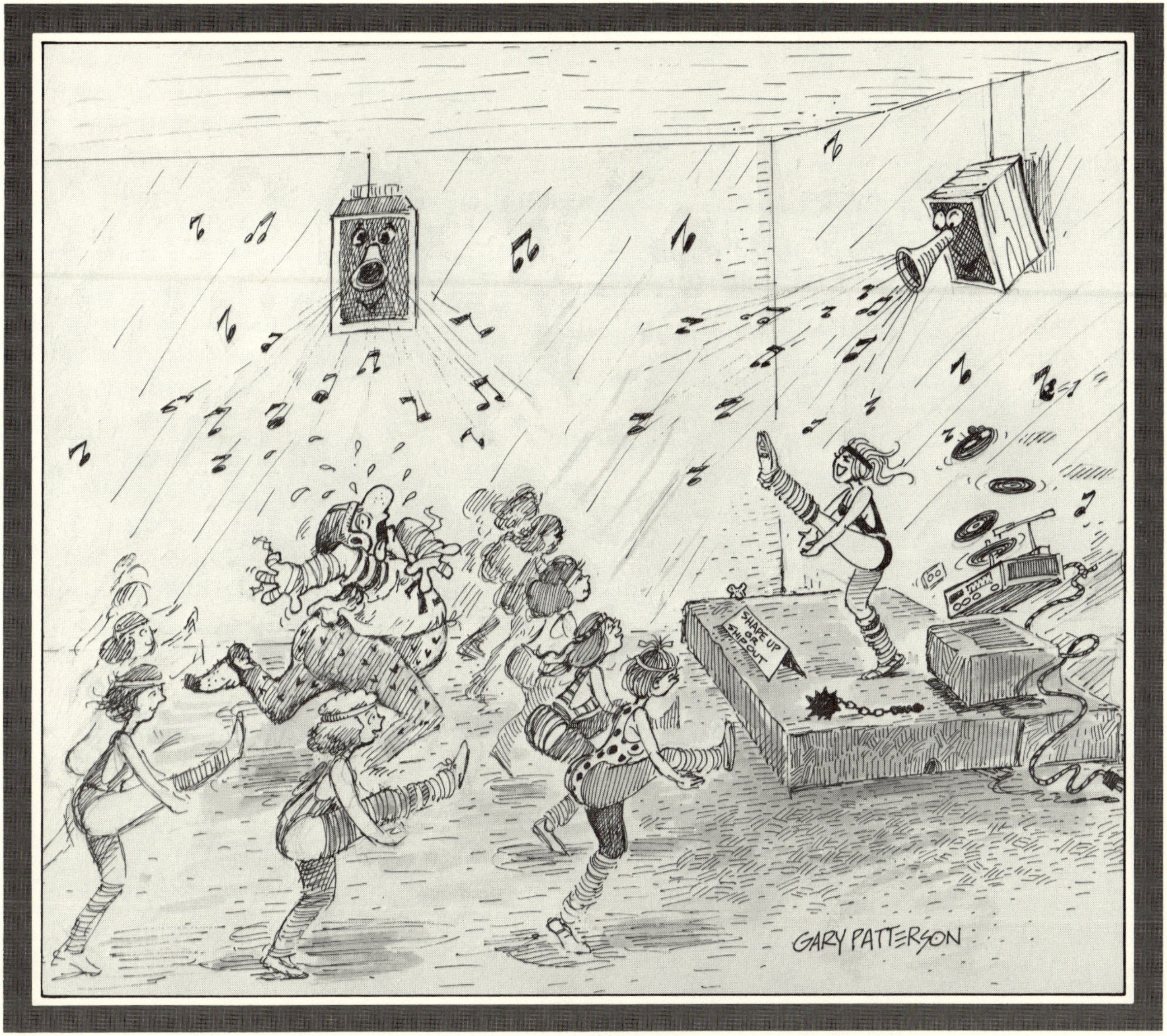

DANCE AEROBICS

DO YOU QUALIFY AS A MAIN-LINE AEROBIC DANCE FANATIC?

1. Which would you rather sleep in? **a.** \$100 pajamas **b.** \$10 night shirt and \$90 leg warmers	**a.** ☐	**b.** ☐
2. Aerobic dance fanatics can never be too thin or have too many shoes.	**TRUE** ☐	**FALSE** ☐
3. Aerobic dance animals don't tell their bodies what they need—their bodies tell them!	**TRUE** ☐	**FALSE** ☐

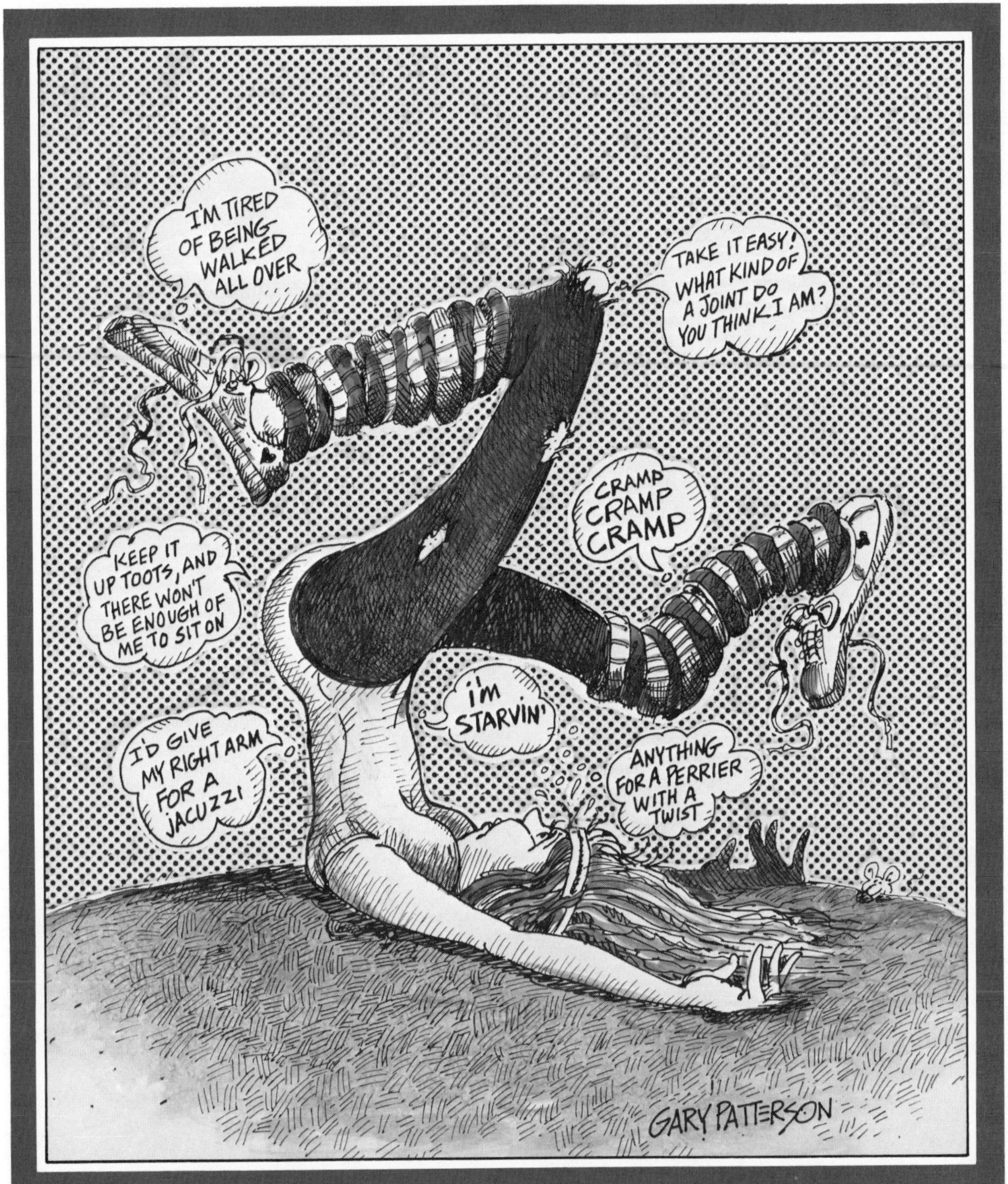
I'M TIRED OF BEING WALKED ALL OVER
TAKE IT EASY! WHAT KIND OF A JOINT DO YOU THINK I AM?
CRAMP CRAMP CRAMP
KEEP IT UP TOOTS, AND THERE WON'T BE ENOUGH OF ME TO SIT ON
I'M STARVIN'
I'D GIVE MY RIGHT ARM FOR A JACUZZI
ANYTHING FOR A PERRIER WITH A TWIST
GARY PATTERSON

SHAPING UP

4. Do you eagerly participate in sexually explicit contortions in a class with strangers that you wouldn't think of doing in bedrooms with lovers?

YES ☐ **NO** ☐ **THE 5TH AMENDMENT** ☐

5. The older aerobic dance fanatics get and the longer they work out, the younger they feel . . . and the older everyone else feels!

TRUE ☐ **FALSE** ☐

6. Are you willing to suffer the agony of hard-core dance aerobics for the ecstacy of what you can do to the rest of us who haven't?

YES ☐ **NO** ☐

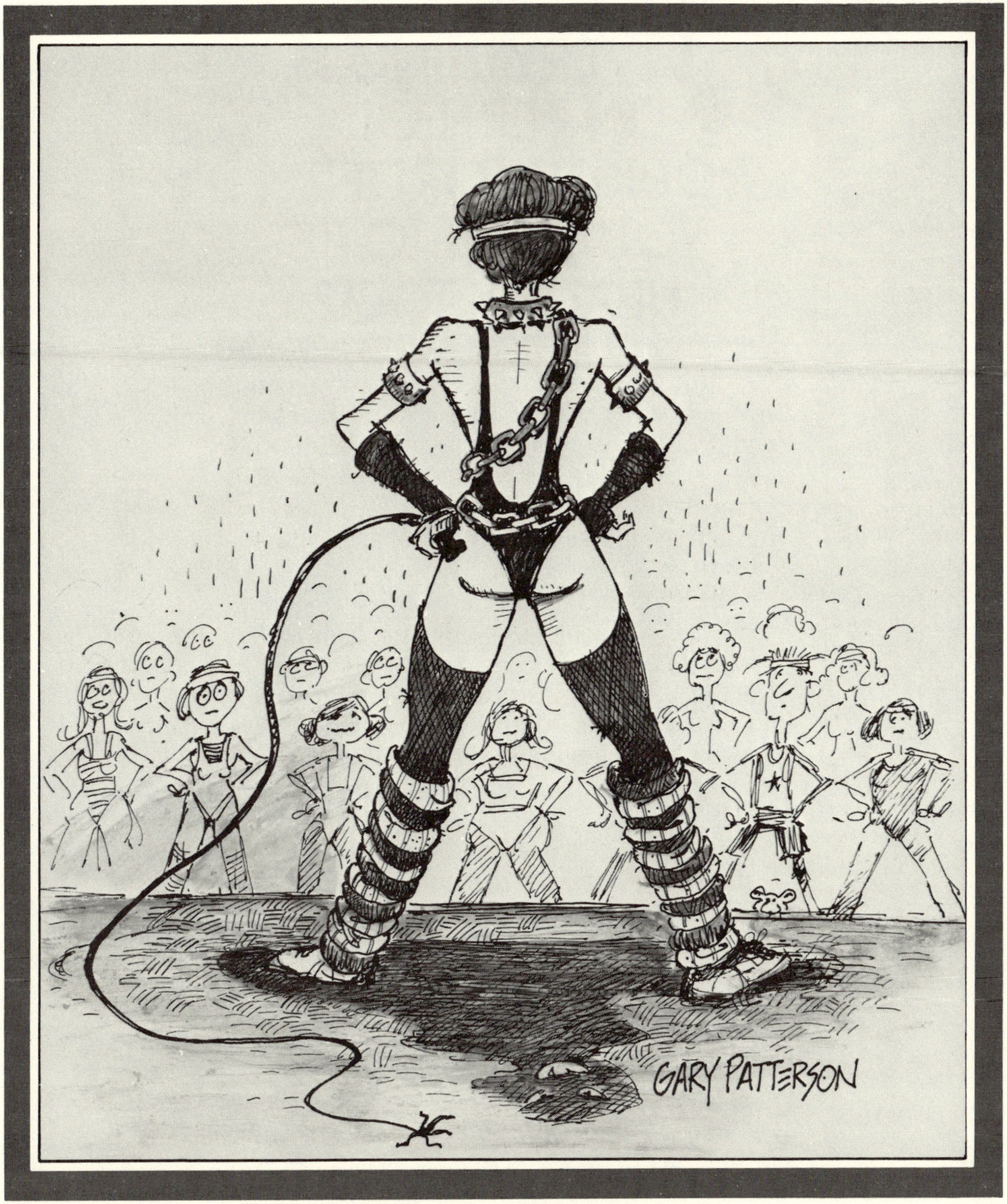

THE DRILL INSTRUCTOR

10
EVERYTHING IS IN PERFECT WORKING ORDER . . . YOU WANT TO BE HEALTHY, TOO?

Within the first couple of months, Aerobic Animals go overboard in their exercising and find themselves looking and feeling more miserable than before they began. This is normal because new Fitness Fanatics think they can change in two weeks what it took them 20 years to achieve.

When it's too late, these walking wounded need the advice of a good doctor. Find a doctor you can relate to on a physical level.

After a thorough examination, a good doctor will advise that given the patient's present exhausted, run down, and altogether woebegone condition, certain tests are needed.

These special "sports physicals" or "stress tests" are specifically designed to tell the doctor whether you are in good enough shape to begin a program of getting in shape.

Stress tests are comprised of such things as stress electrocardiograms, blood profiles, strength/flexibility tests, lung function efficiency, and—the ultimate stress test—reading the bill while standing up without falling down.

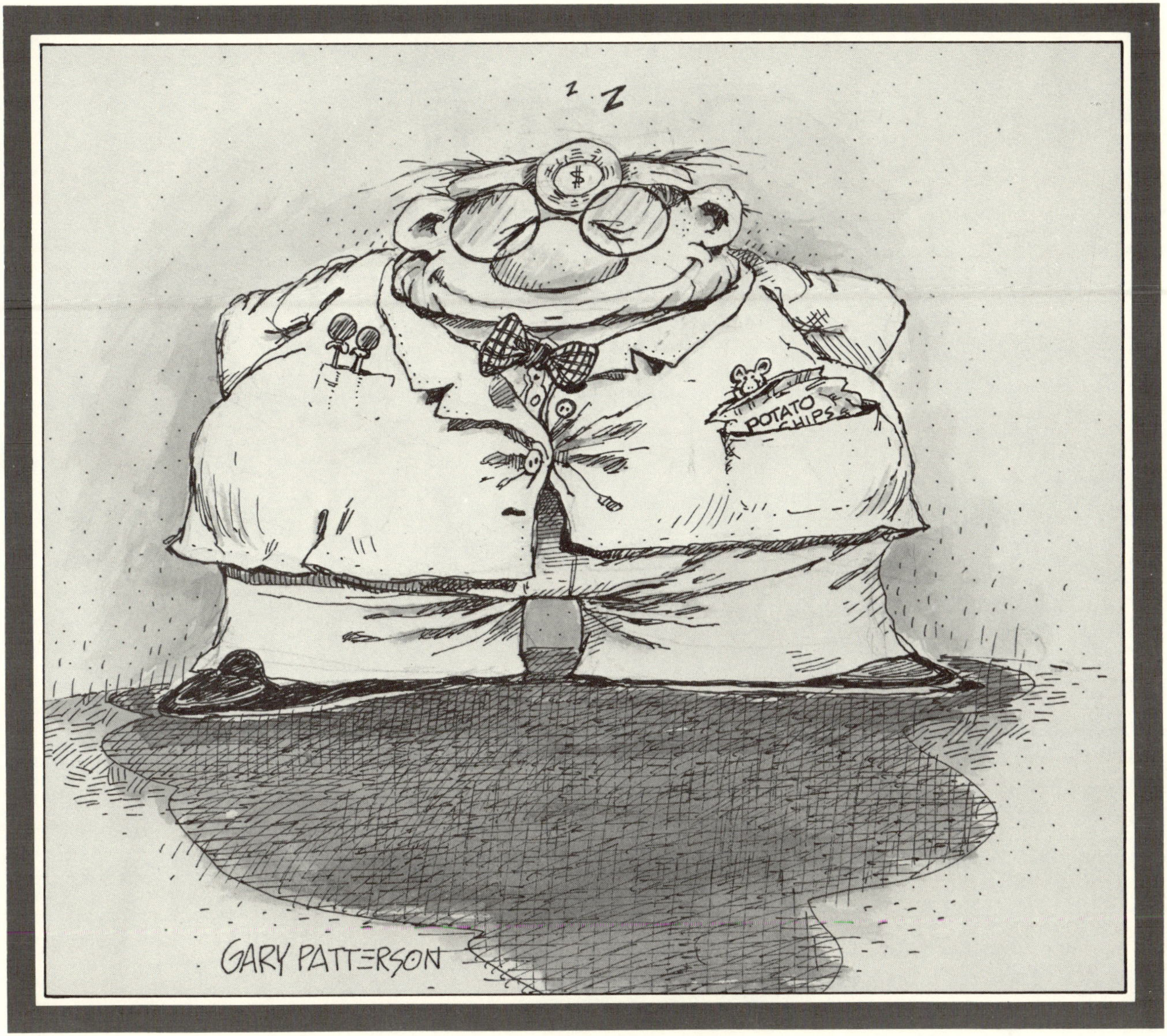

THE GOOD DOCTOR

PART II

The Muscle Hustle

Fitness Fanatics believe working out is a lot more enjoyable at a health club, where fun and congeniality is as much a part of working out as working out.

There is a big difference between the kind of people who go to places that use words like "health" and "fitness" and "spa" in their names and those real bodybuilders who prefer to pump iron at places that go by a man's first name followed by the word "gym"—as in Otto's Gym or Rocky's Rocks.

A real bodybuilder would never be caught working out in a place with a name like Elmer's Fitness Spa and Health Food Oasis.

Run-of-the-treadmill fitness enthusiasts are more comfortable, however, in a looser, less disciplined environment.

The biggest difference between gyms and fitness clubs is that the hunks and hunkettes who go to bodybuilding gyms spend a lot of time looking at themselves in mirrors, checking out definition and separation of lats, abs, traps, hams, pecs . . .

The folks who go to the fitness spas spend more time checking out *everyone else's* hams, pecs, gluteus maximus, etc.

11

TIME FOR A NEW WAIST DISPOSAL SYSTEM?

Health and fitness clubs are great places for the undergraduate Fitness Fanatic to submerge themselves in the world of would-be lean, hard bodies.

The following is a general guide to aid in making the decision whether it's really time to consider a new waist disposal system.

- You are probably not in as good shape as you could be if you can put your bra on backwards and it fits better.
- Your vitality and stamina are not what they should be if you have to sit down to brush your teeth.
- You are probably eating more than your body requires if you grab a quick bite at McDonald's and the manager has to change the numbers on the sign outside.

FOOD FOR THOUGHT

Freud said, "Being entirely honest with oneself is good exercise." Admitting how much you hate exercising is the best exercise of all!

12

FUN AND GAMES AT THE NEIGHBORHOOD HEALTH CLUB

The hot and heavy action of the singles bar has moved into the jacuzzi of the neighborhood fitness spa. This is the real hot spot in town, where men and women of all ages can go and pick up on some heavy breathing action.

From the moment you join a health club you must look like you know what you're doing.

Men should always walk around with a thick leather lifting belt buckled securely around their middle. You must look like a bodybuilder even if you're only trying to hold up your underwear.

There is a certain glow and animal magnetism to a body that is dripping in good honest sweat, but that doesn't mean you have to get crazy. A quick shower *before* working out, then putting your tank-top and shorts on and drip-drying as you stroll around the exercise room is sure to get you the same admiring glances that busting your guts has.

It usually isn't too long before newcomers to the club get excited about working out on the latest weight machines. You quickly learn that the secret of mastering these machines is not how much iron you can pump, but how many agonized expressions you can screw up on your face.

As the Fitness Fanatic becomes more committed to a regular schedule of exercising, you learn how to breathe properly—or die of strangulation. Slowly you make the transition from between-the-teeth inhaling and expelling through pursed lips, to real open-glottis air sucking and exhaling like an active steel mill.

But the best part of working out in the friendly atmosphere of a spa is the one-on-one competition.

Two people often find themselves working out on opposite sides of the same piece of equipment. The more heart-felt gasps from one side fuel the competitive fires back on the other side and before long the two Fitness Fanatics vie to see who can outgrunt the other. This usually lasts until you notice that while you are gasping and groaning with one hundred and fifty pounds, your competitor is gutting up only fifteen.

It is then that the "good-time" Fitness Fanatic may decide it's a good time to get in shape for something easy, like the Boston Marathon.

13

GETTING "RIPPED" AT BRUNO'S GYM

At places like Bruno's—not Elmer's—bodies glisten and glow with the Chanel No. 5 of a real bodybuilder's gym—sweat.

Unlike other Fitness Fanatics, true bodybuilders are a bit old-fashioned in their loyalty to free weights. No fancy cam-type equipment for them. They prefer to grunt it out with a couple of dumbbells.

They usually work out with friends, rooting them on to greater feats of strength and endurance. When they are too exhausted to make even one more rep, their partner will exhort them onward with cries of:

> "C'mon, one more time. Push, push, push!
> You can do it. C'mon, c'mon, c'mon!
> One more, more, more, ONE MORE!!"

And when they do it, the partner will smile and say:

> "I lied. Give me one more."

Really incredible hulks work out with barbells so heavy it takes two to lift the bar into position so one hulk can play with it.

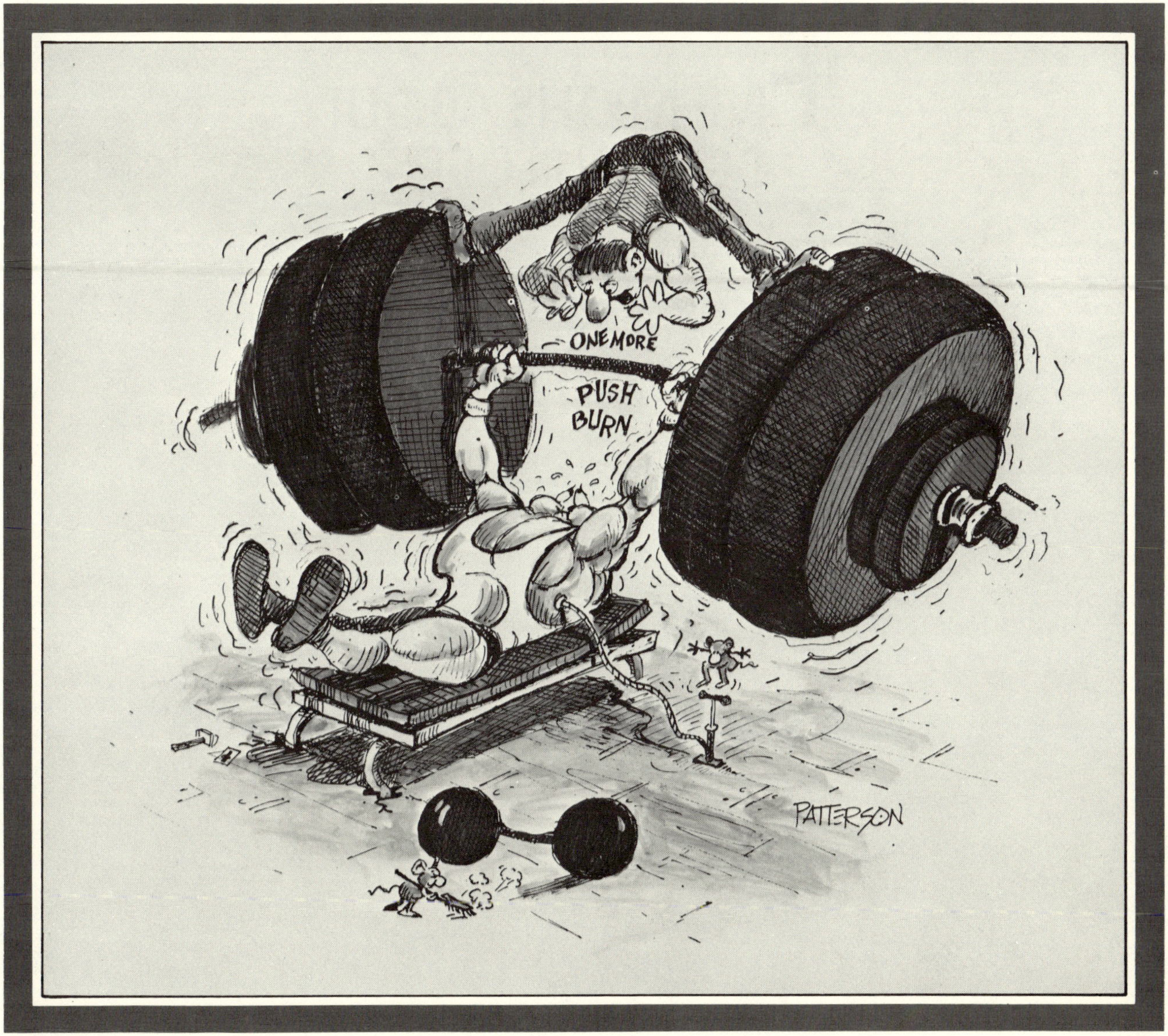

THE INCREDIBLE HULK

14

FIVE MYTHS ABOUT BODYBUILDERS

It is high time we exploded a few myths about those mega-muscled hunks and hunkettes who look like they've migrated from the planet Popeye.

MYTH #1

Bodybuilders are airheads.

FALSE!

Just because their body parts and muscle groups go beyond the world of known measurement and make their heads look tiny, that does not mean there is nothing up there. Remember, they are not the ones looking for overnight diets and fancy machines to whip them magically into shape.

We *are the ones* eager *to sell our souls and mortgage our mothers to find out their "secrets" so we can look like that in a month and a half.*

MYTH #2

Bodybuilders walk around with their arms away from their sides because of their incredibly developed triceps and latissimus dorsi.

NOT SO!

The truth is that if they ever let their arms hang down close to their sides, the incredible suction created in their crater-like pits would make it impossible ever to lift their arms back up again.

MYTH #3

Hunks and hunkettes wear clothing three sizes too small to make their muscles look three times as big.

UNTRUE!

They paint their clothes on.

MYTH #4

Bodybuilders are vain and narcissistic.

PATENTLY RIDICULOUS!

Bodybuilders are the first to say they are just like everyone else—only more so. In fact, most of them used to look like most of us. Bodybuilders resolutely believe that anyone can look like they do if they will just try to think of their bodies as a giant piece of rock. Chisel away the rough edges and inside all of us lives the granite physique of Hercules waiting to flex. And being stoned helps.

MYTH #5

If really musclebound people stop working out, their muscles will turn to fat.

FALSE, FALSE, FALSE!!

Use it or lose it.

FOOD FOR THOUGHT

You should be very careful about the oils you use in cooking. There are good oils and evil oils.

Olive oil is good. If it doesn't suit your taste, you can always rub it all over your body and pose!

15

THE HARDWARE OF HARD BODIES

True Fitness Fanatics use only the best equipment. Staying in top physical shape requires staying on top of the latest in the hardware of hard bodies.

Over the last few years, manufacturers of exercise equipment have become convinced that Fitness Fanatics and would-be Fitness Fanatics will buy whichever hardware promises to give them the best body in the shortest possible time with the least amount of suffering.

Of course they are right—which probably explains why every other week there is a new apparatus on the market that guarantees to do something to your body in half the time the old equipment promised. That the old equipment lied doesn't shake your confidence in the new paraphernalia.

These new high-tech, computerized machines have tremendous appeal, particularly to those half-hearted enthusiasts who won't admit it in public, but secretly feel they have worked too hard for too many years to get where they are, to now work out even harder to get back to the way they were!

They would much rather put in a daily routine of EXER-CUSE: That's one part exercise to three parts excuses for not doing it.

But because even that one part exercise is more than they really want to endure, they are constantly looking for any piece of equipment that will magically transform their bods into gods. The high cost of these machines is no object. These people know whatever they do is going to hurt. The question is where: their arches or their MasterCard/VISA.

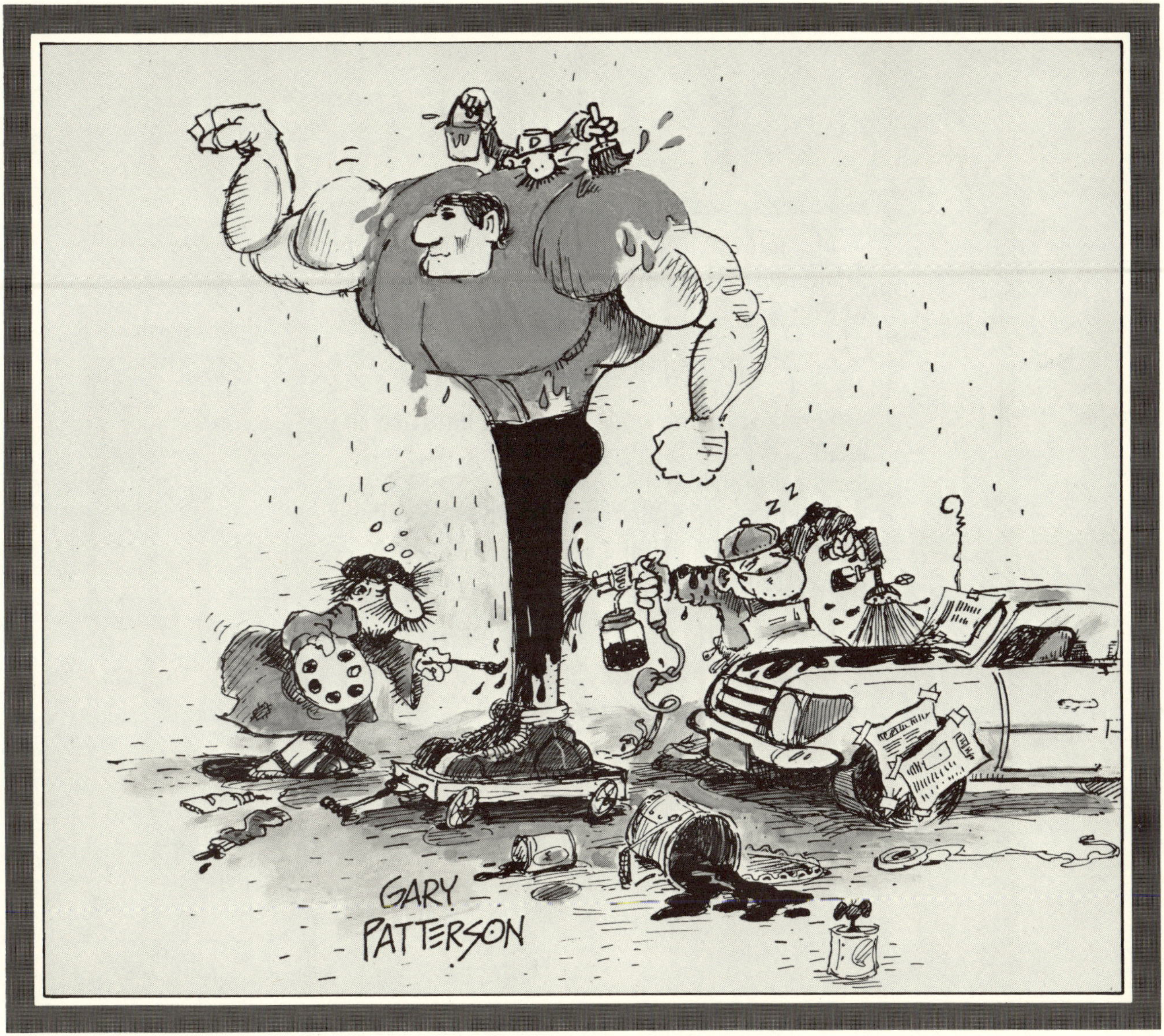

THE BODYBUILDER

The following is an overview of the most advanced in aerobic, strength training, body toning and conditioning hardware available:

ROWING MACHINES

The best of these allow you to capture the total body exhilaration of rowing without keeping your oar in.

Even the cheaper machines have a stroke counter which usually counts up to 999. After that, *you* have the stroke.

STATIONARY BICYCLES

High-tech stationary bikes are wonderful achievements in the application of computer technology to health and fitness. Hop on one of these magnificent cycles, pedal your gastrocnemiuses into mush, and watch the computerized dashboard interface your mileage, elapsed time, calories burned per hour, work performed in watts, pulse rate, blood pressure, date of birth, your astrological forecast, and the weather in Toledo in one byte!

SCALES

Every fitness enthusiast should keep a sharp eye on weight. An accurate scale is an absolute must.

One of the best and most expensive types is the balance-beam scale like those used in doctors' offices. The top-of-the-line balance beam scales make use of bubble leveling devices and fiber optic electronic indicators to double check the counterweights for perfect balance.

You could also save a bundle and hop on the check-out scale at the local grocery store.

Scales are advertised as either having "cast iron bases for a lifetime of rugged use," or "all steel construction made to stand up under years of repeated stress." But remember, they only come with a 90-day warranty.

And then there is the scale that actually talks:

> "Your weight is two hundred and fifty-seven pounds. Up three pounds, six ounces from yesterday. Have a nice day!"

Now that's the scale you want to kick the springs out of, on a scale of 1 to 1 ton.

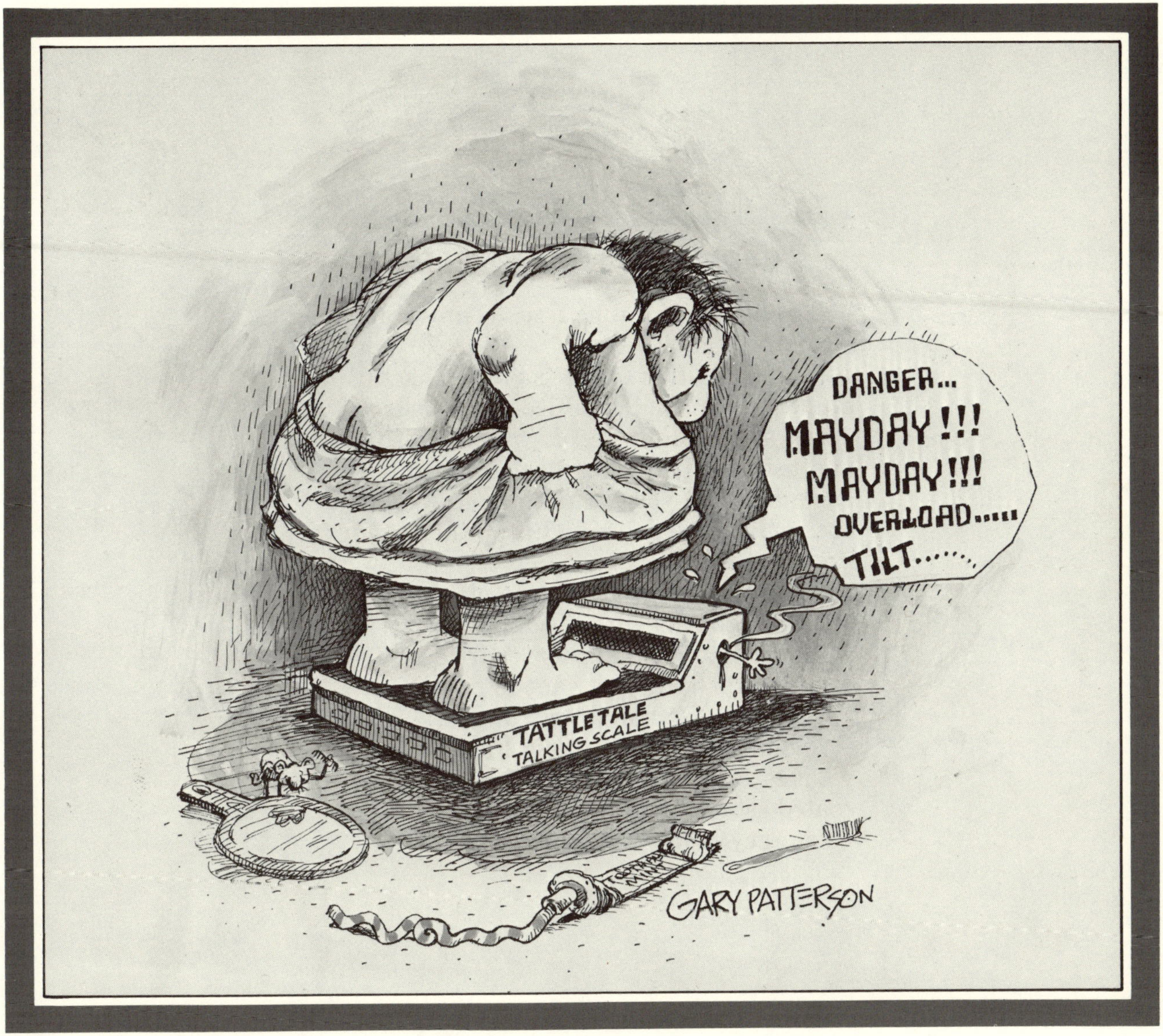
DANGER...
MAYDAY!!!
MAYDAY!!!
OVERLOAD.....
TILT......
TATTLE TALE
TALKING SCALE
GARY PATTERSON

WEIGHING IN

BARBELLS AND DUMBBELLS

Barbell and dumbbell sets come in all sizes and styles.

A new addition to the traditional set of dumbbells is small, padded dumbbells. These are good for people who are also small and padded. These dumbbells are soft enough that if you get tired from working out, you can lie down and prop them under each ear for pillows.

However, in most cases, an old-fashioned set of dumbbells with black cast iron weights is an ideal starter—particularly if you aren't sure if you want to pump anything more than a tank of gas.

The more serious Fitness Fanatic may want to spend a little more for a rubber-coated set of weights that soften the blow when they land on your toes.

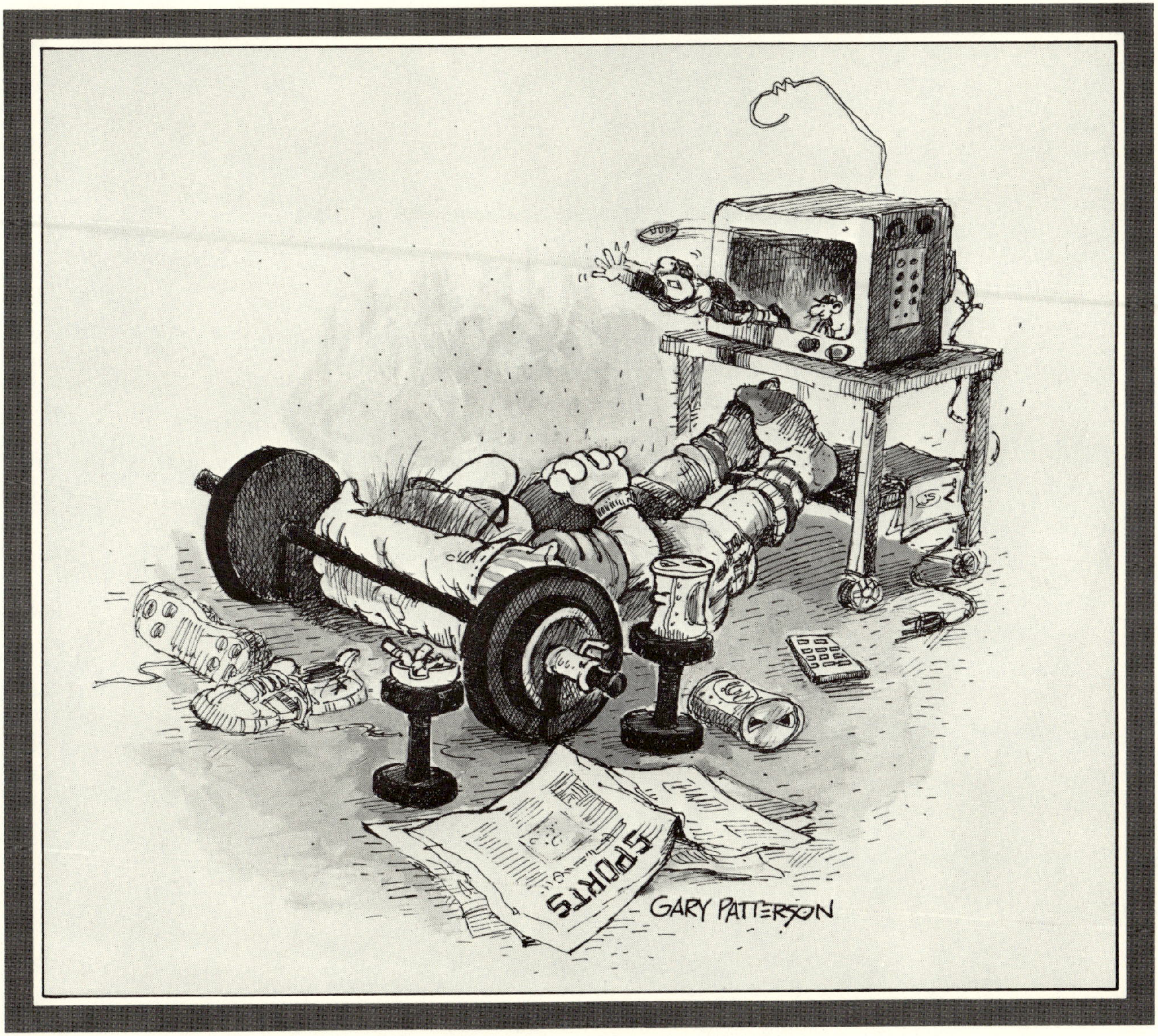

THE SERIOUS WEIGHT LIFTER

TREADMILLS

The state of the art in treadmills for jogging and running surpasses that of even the most high-tech computerized bikes. Today's sophisticated motor-powered treadmill is designed and built to duplicate the exact conditions you experience in the real world.

Why give up bad weather, traffic, air pollution, potholes, and police dogs when you can have them all in the privacy and comfort of your home or office?

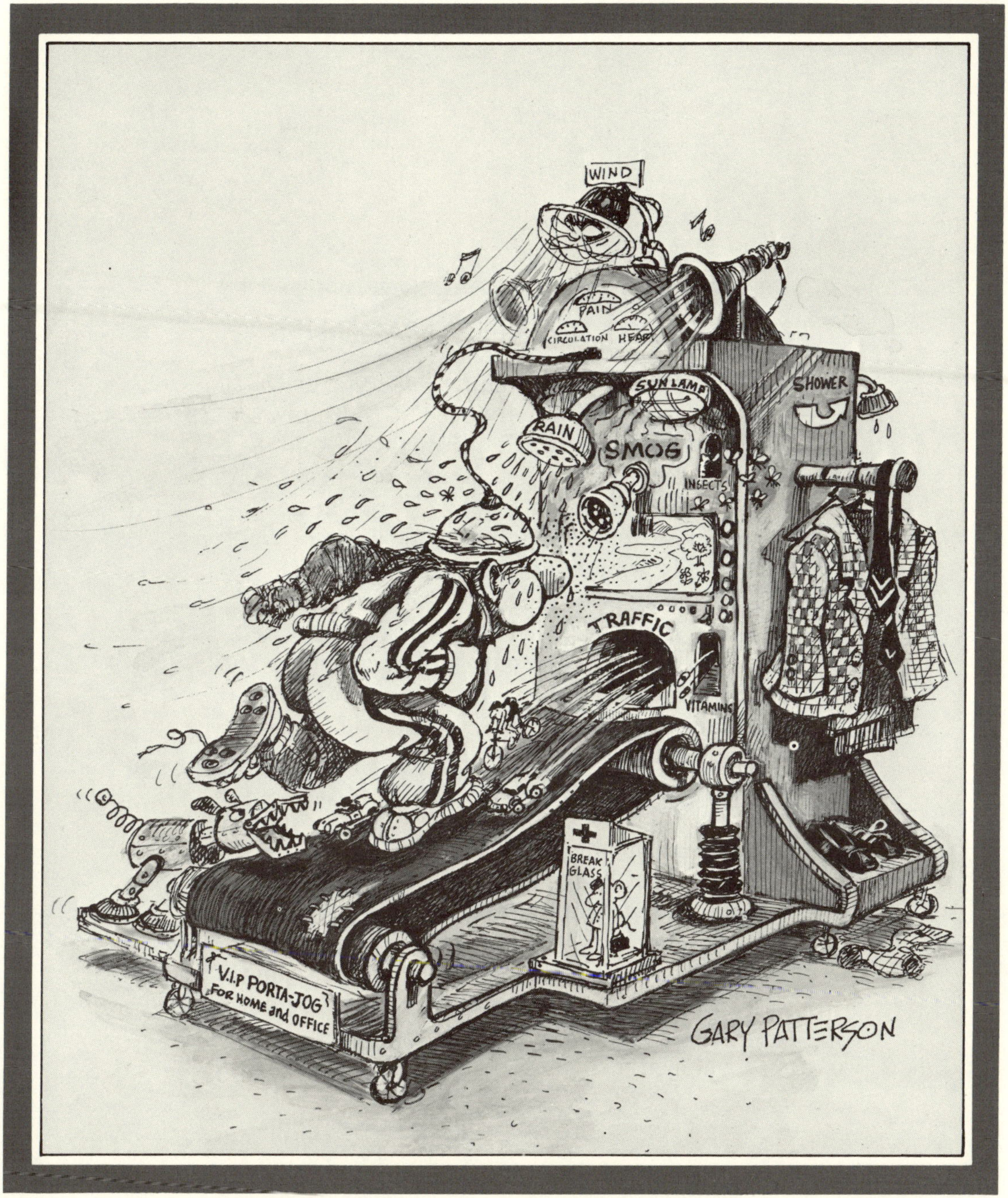

STATE-OF-THE-ART TREADMILL

WEIGHT TRAINING MACHINES

"Conditioning and toning." Whatever that means nobody will tell you, but there are catalogs full of exotic equipment guaranteeing to do it to your body faster and easier than the next piece of hardware.

Some of this equipment makes use of your own body weight for resistance. You're "conditioned and toned" by pulling yourself up and down inclined rails on a glide board. How hard you work out is determined by the steepness of the board and the size of your hard-earned assets on it. Lightweight and portable, the equipment is strong enough to accommodate you, even if you're not.

Probably more popular are the heavyweight multiposition machines that make use of hydraulic cylinders, steel coil springs, or traditional weight stacks.

These machines are designed and marketed to appeal to the primordial beast, the Fitness Fanatic. These machines do very well with third-string hockey players, encyclopedia salespeople, and IRA fighters.

RUNNERS' WATCHES

High-tech stopwatches are a must for the serious runner.

The morning of a big race an alarm wakes you up and a microlight in the LCD panel displays the day, date, and year—before you open your eyes.

The gun sounds and you're off. Press a button. A mile into the race you press it again and the watch computes and projects your finish time. You run faster. Even if you're still in bed.

Another mile and an alarm signals your pace has slowed. You pick up the pace like an Olympic champion. Press another button and the watch displays your maximum oxygen uptake and pulse rate, and reserves a bed for you at the hospital.

These watches are guaranteed to run that extra mile—even if you can't.

GRAVITY INVERSION EXERCISERS

Your body wages constant war with gravity. Your organs sag. Your skin droops. Gravity inversion devices counteract this law of nature by swinging the body upside down, allowing organs to sag back up and double chins to become drooping foreheads.

The mounting evidence in support of hanging by your heels is hard to dispute. When was the last time you saw a fat bat with a bad back?

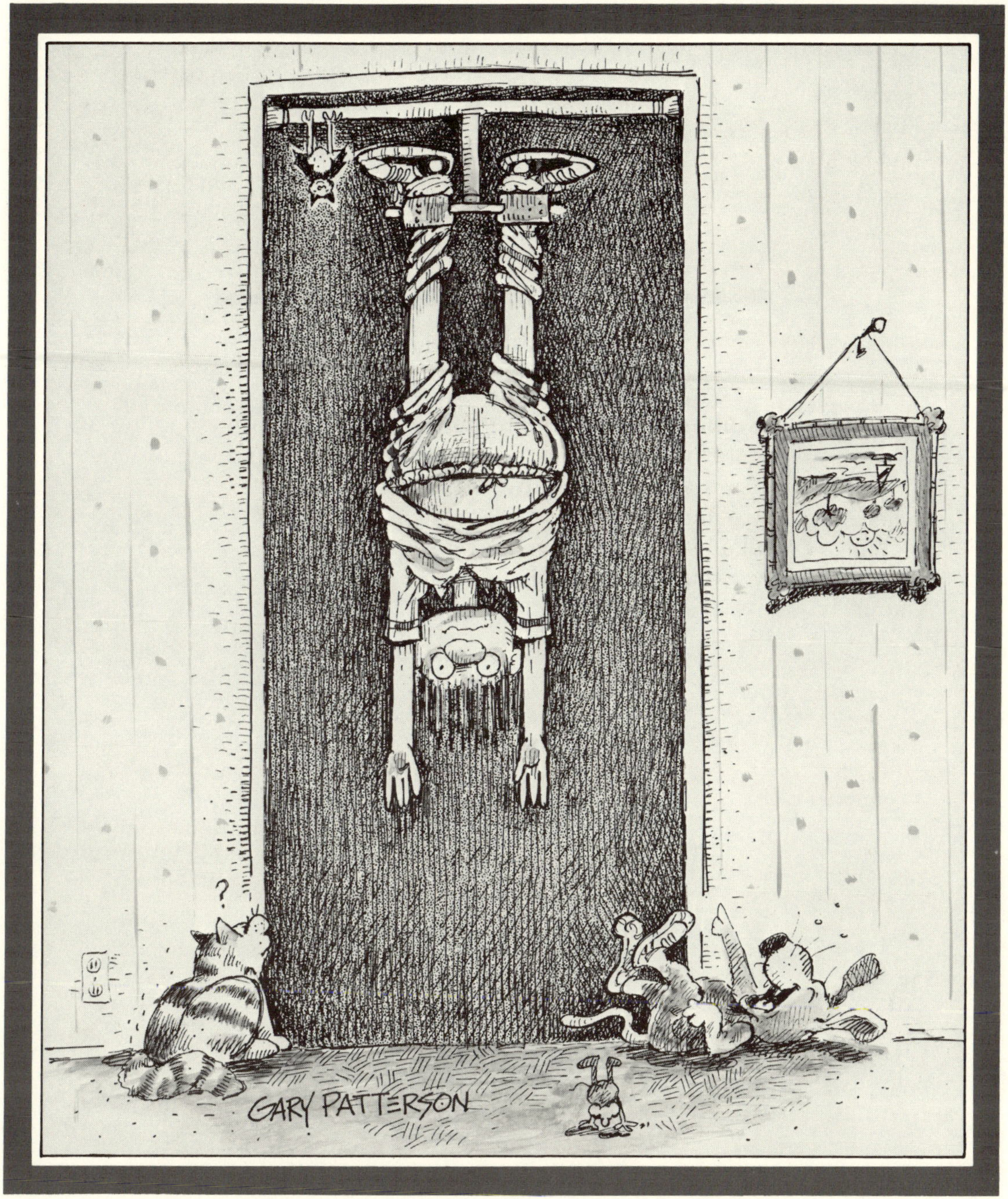
?
GARY PATTERSON

MINITRAMPOLINES

Bouncing, twisting, kicking, or rope-skipping on a minitrampoline gives you better coordination, balance, and agility. It also makes you jumpy.

What's best about them is that you can take them anywhere and get a quick workout—even on the elevator.

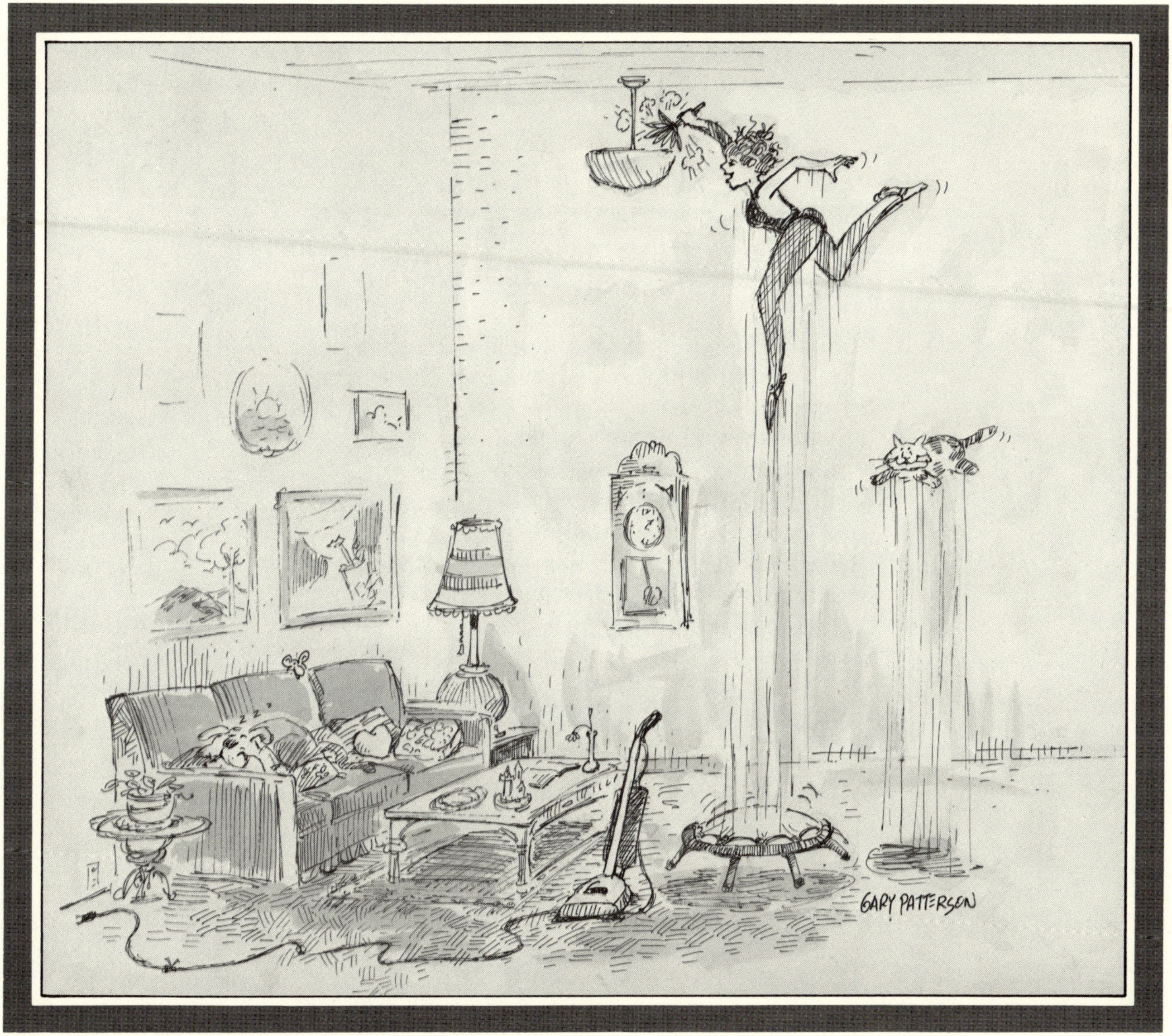
GARY PATTERSON

VARIABLE RESISTANCE CAM MACHINES

Sold under a variety of trade names, these cam machines have revolutionized the fitness movement. Fitness Fanatics get all pumped up about working out on them.

The only drawback is that they promise such incredible results with so little effort that people who buy them go out to the garage three times a week and fondle the hardware—figuring they can osmose their bodies into incredible hulks.

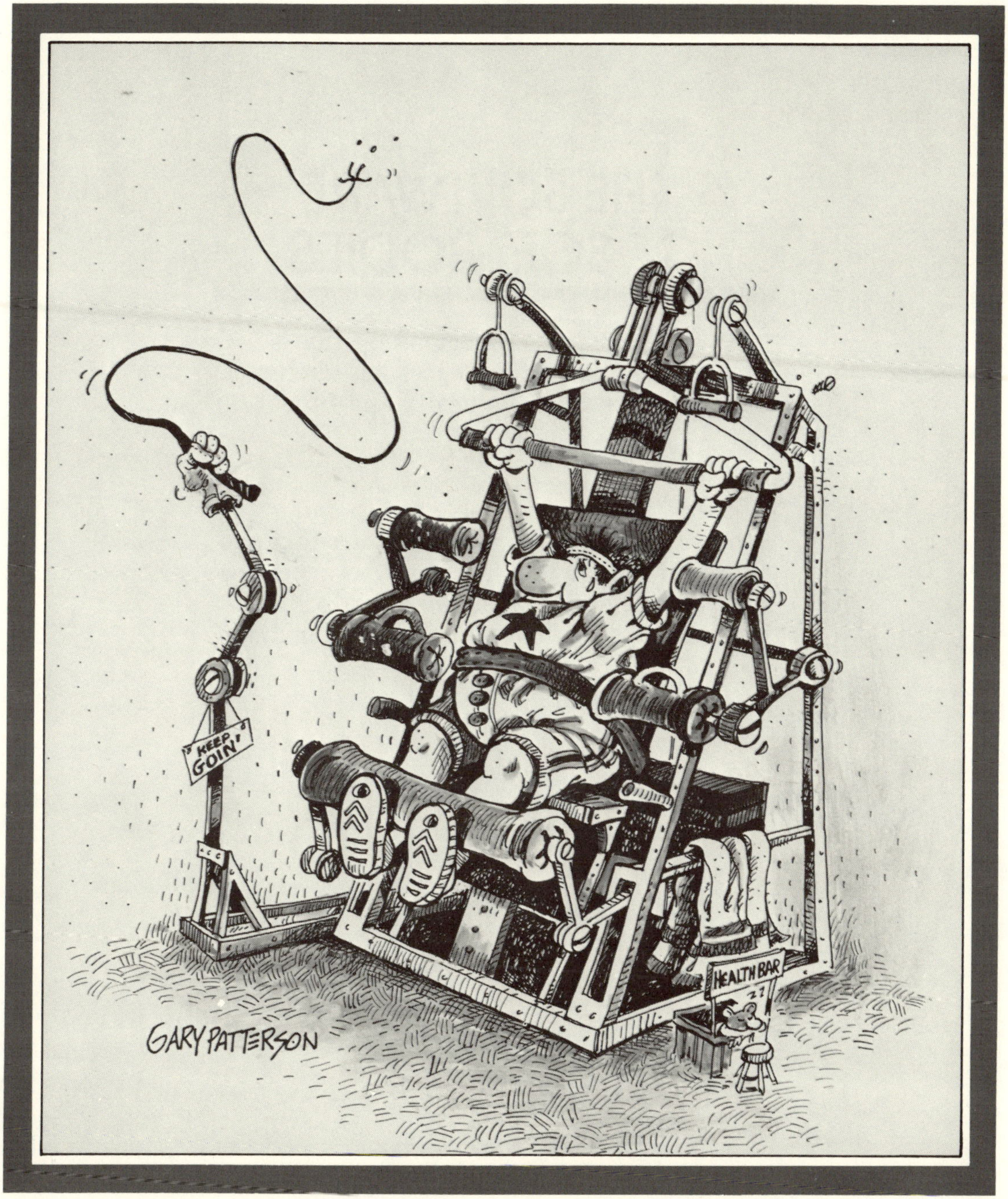

WORK THAT BODY

16

THE SOFTWARE OF SOFT BODIES

Anybody who has ever run for a bus or accidentally touched their toes has written a book or made a tape on health and fitness.

BOOKS

Most of the big expensive health and fitness books by TV and movie stars take the approach of showing the reader how they too can turn themselves from an ugly duckling into a swan, just the way the superstar did.

You can tell how serious a movie star is about fitness by the way he or she dedicates the book:

I would like to dedicate this book and give special thanks to:

Miss Twinky, my co-star and ever-ready partner in couples exercises.

My lawyer, who did such a great job with my divorce.

Paco, for keeping my hair from falling out.

Mr. Max, for keeping my face and skin natural with never more than an hour in make-up.

My dental hygienist, for keeping my gums pink and happy.

My stunt-double, for lifting the really heavy weights until I could step in for the last rep.

The tanning machine, for giving me that golden glow.

There are also books by those women who have exercise shows on TV at 5:30 every morning. They usually start something like this:

> Guess what? I've gone and written my very own book by staying up till 6 P.M. each night.

Books by professional dancers, who really know the hard work and sacrifice necessary to be in shape to go on every night, are popular.

> Are dancers born that way?
> YES!
> The rest of you will just have to buy my book and bust your buns.

Then there are also hundreds of small paperbacks that guarantee to *Flatten Your Stomach in Seven Days or Your Botticelli Belly Back!*.

And then there's *Thin Thighs in Thirty Minutes*, with a picture of people who never had thighs to begin with—unlike the authors.

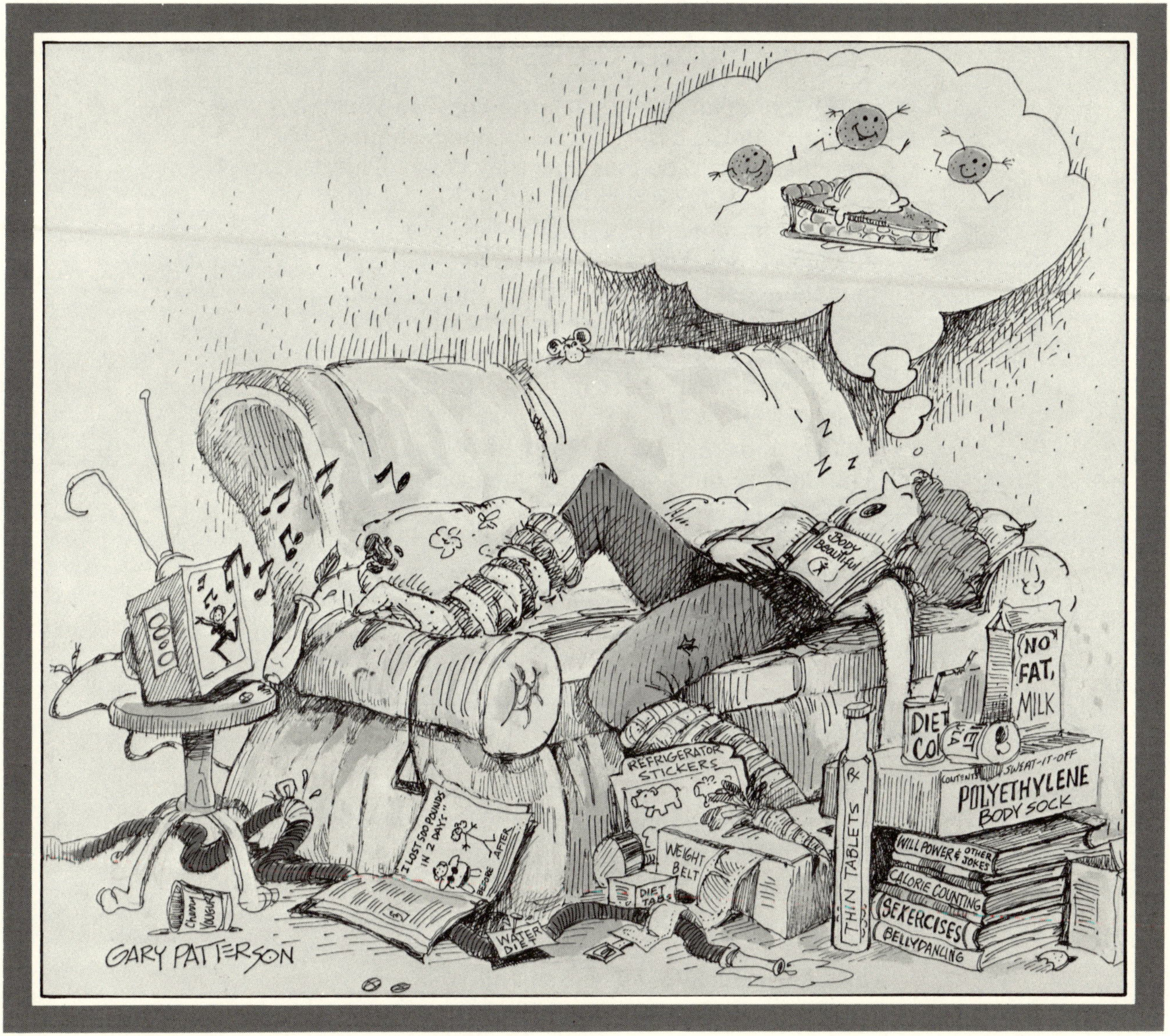
Body Beautiful
NO FAT, MILK
DIET CO
SWEAT-IT-OFF
CONTENTS
POLYETHYLENE BODY SOCK
REFRIGERATOR STICKERS
WEIGHT BELT
THIN TABLETS
WILL POWER & OTHER JOKES
CALORIE COUNTING
SEXERCISES
BELLYDANCING
I LOST 500 POUNDS IN 2 DAYS"
BEFORE
AFTER
DIET TABS
WATER DIET
GARY PATTERSON

VIDEO CASSETTES

Now you can have bootcamp right in your living room! A drill instructor has a shape-up video that is as tough as they come. This cassette isn't for everyone, but drill instructors don't care. They're looking for a few good men and women who are willing to put their behinds on the firing line.

And there are exercise cassettes by the Queen of Conditioning, the High Priestess of Perspiration, the Barishnikov of Butt Burners!

This actress wants us to believe that if she can do it at her age, then you can, too.

WRONG!

We can't keep up with her, but neither can anyone else.

This woman is not like the rest of us. Her muscles, flesh, and bones are made of silly putty. She does things with her body parts that should be censored, and her tape ought to be rated Rx. No one should be allowed to buy or rent one without a written prescription from their doctor.

And that fabulous smile! It never stops for 90 minutes. Anyone who can smile through the ordeal she puts herself through is an actress of staying power. Give her an Oscar and maybe she'll move on to something else less hazardous to our coffee and rolls, especially the ones around the stomach.

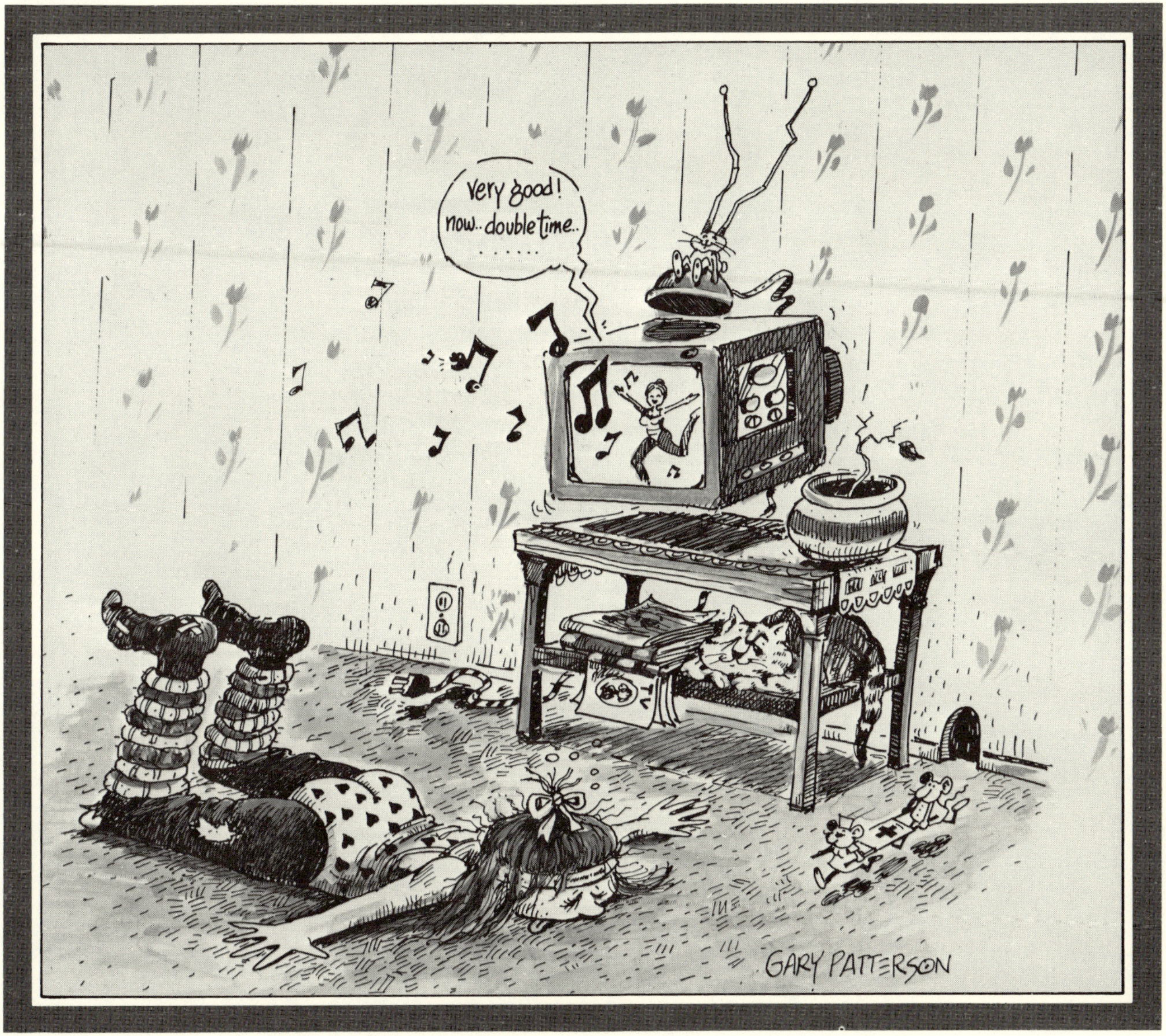

HOME FITNESS

STUFF IN MAGAZINES

The mail order software available in fitness and bodybuilding magazines costs an arm and a leg. Send away for some of the stuff offered by former Mr. Universes, Mr. Olympias, and the Triple Crown Filly of Flex Appeal, and your letter carrier's body will be at risk.

These famous bodybuilders have got everything you need! Courses for building massive arms, a wide powerful back, doorway-wide shoulders, legs of an oak, and your own personal training bag with heavy-duty straps to take the weight of all the rest of the stuff you're going to buy—the *really important* stuff like: T-shirts, tank tops, posing trunks, and more!

FOOD FOR THOUGHT

"Never eat more than you can lift."

—Miss Piggy

17

THE UNDER-WEAR OF EVERY BODY

The Golden Rule for beginning Fitness Fanatics:

> "Accentuate the positive, camouflage the negative, latch on to a color that's hot, and hang around the juice bar looking liquid."

When it comes to exercise apparel, there is something for every body:

- Bikinis for men and women of every physique. Brief-cut suits for brief-cut bodies. Full-cut suits with contoured seats for full-cut pople with contoured seats.
- Trunks with a tapered front and no rear seam if you have no rear seam. And trunks with high-cut sides and 3-piece seats for bodybuilders with 3-piece seats. We're talking buns!

- There's also flab-fighting underwear made of rubber that traps natural body heat and promotes instant perspiration. Wear it at home, at work. In seconds the body begins melting away excess water and fat. Comes with matching golashes and mop.
- Real bodybuilders wear whatever they feel like! Ripped T-shirts go with ripped bodies, which is bodybuilding talk for being really shredded, bodybuilding talk for being built like Godzilla.
- Joggers wear $300 warmup suits—but only for grocery shopping.
- Real runners stick to shorts over sweatpants. They've never stopped running long enough to earn $300!

18
IF THE SHOE FITS . . . IT'LL PROBABLY COST YOU AN ARM AND A LEG

The types and styles of running shoes are also endless, which is really not surprising when you consider that fifty million Americans own running shoes. Of course, fewer than twenty million actually run—and most of those only when trying to keep up with a member of the opposite sex.

The strides in running shoe design are lapping the rest of the sports field. There is a computerized running shoe in development that will actually talk to the runner. A computer chip in the midsole records all the data about your run. When you finish, you remove the shoe and attach it to your home computer. Your computer screen reads out everything about your run: number of steps, force of impact, miles covered, speed. In some cases, the computer has been known to break out in a cold sweat.

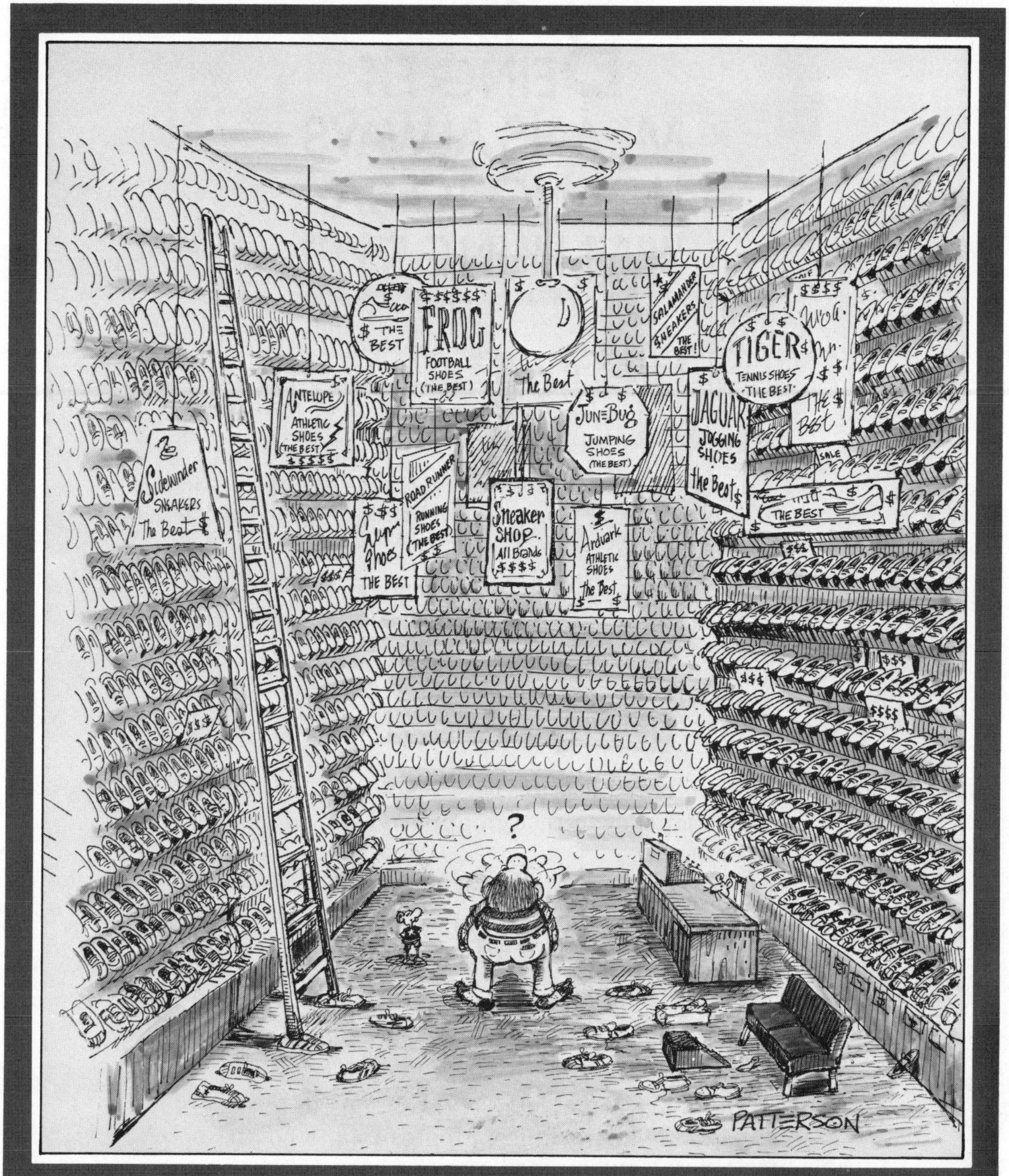

DECISIONS, DECISIONS

19
BEING FIT MEANS ALWAYS HAVING TO SAY, "I'M HUNGRY!"

Being incredibly fit and constantly hungry means you're a Fitness Fanatic. History records many famous physical fitness nuts who had insatiable appetites.

Julius Caesar could never get enough salad or whipped orange drinks. Et tu, Brutus.

Attila the Hun's full name was really Attila the Hungry. The man ate like an elephant.

Confucius ate fortune cookies by the bushel—and got most of his material that way.

Sir Isaac Newton was a closet figaholic, even though apples dropped on his head.

The great lawyer, politician, and master of the English tongue, Francis Bacon, had a thing for bagels, cream cheese, and tongue.

And of course, William Shakespeare, had a thing for Bacon.

There are some notable exceptions to the rule. Take, for instance, Montezuma, who ate *too much* Mexican food and has been taking out his revenge on the rest of us ever since.

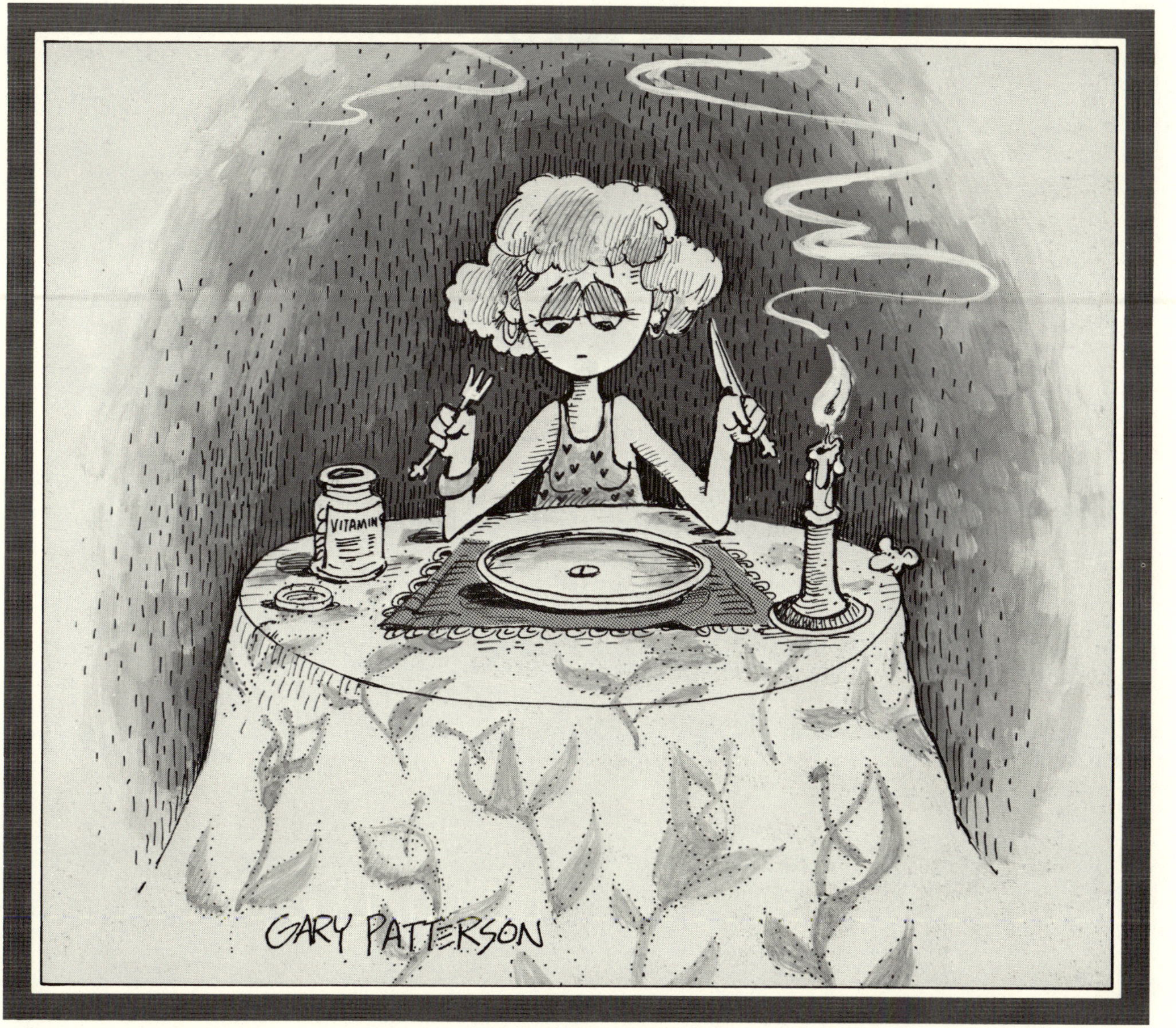

BON APPETIT

20

IS THERE A FITNESS FANATIC IN YOUR LIFE?

Fitness Fanatics are a mixed bag, but some are more committed than others—many ought to be.

Some are willing to bite the bean sprouts and pay the price for health and fitness. Others prefer to make it easier on themselves with time payments—usually interest only. If six months later they haven't reduced their balance, they don't care. They feel comfortable with their assets right where they are.

All of which brings us to the bottom line: How can you tell if someone near or dear to you is really a Fitness Fanatic, or merely a pretender to the title?

- With real Fitness Fanatics there are no ifs, ands, or butts. They work out according to schedule come rain or come shine, for richer or poorer, in sickness and in health, in this life and the NEXT!
- The only time they wear the latest in fitness fashions is when it's their own design: torn sweatshirt and ragged shorts.
- These people worship their *own* bodies the way other people worship *other* people's bodies.
- They don't know the meaning of the words wet noodle arms, frog butt hips, and cottage cheese thighs. They also don't know the meaning of the words Pepperidge Farms Deep Dish Danish.

Fitness Fanatics are a hazard to everybody else's well-being! The carnage of pot bellies, sagging fannies, and tidal wave thighs wasted away in the wake of a Fitness Fanatic's crusade is often nothing less than a criminal violation against the faint of heart and weak of knee—the very people who made this great country what it is today!

The fitter than thou, the healthier than hell, would do well to remember the immortal words on the Statue of Liberty:

"Give me your tired, YOUR HUNGRY,
your huddled masses. . . ."

Nobody said anything about being dynamic, vivacious, well-nourished, and disgustingly cheerful.

If there's a Fitness Fanatic in your life, run for it.

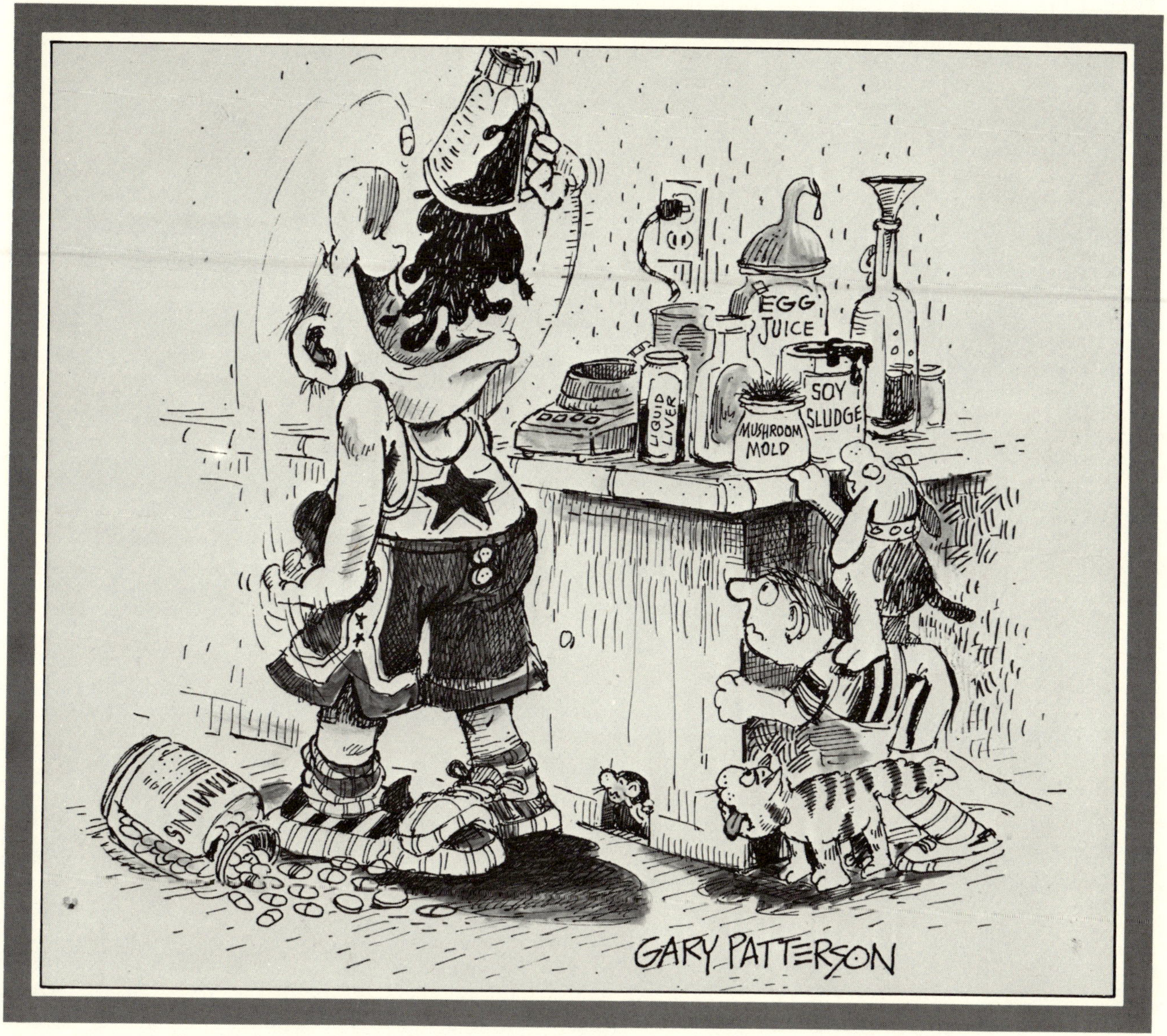

IS THERE A FITNESS FANATIC IN YOUR LIFE?